# Therapeutics in Respiratory Disease

*For Churchill Livingstone*

*Publisher:* Mike Parkinson
*Project Editor:* Dilys Jones
*Copy Editor:* Thérèse Duriez
*Production Controller:* Debra Barrie
*Sales Promotion Executive:* Duncan Jones

# Therapeutics in Respiratory Disease

## Peter J. Barnes MA DM DSc FRCP
Professor of Thoracic Medicine, National Heart and Lung Institute; Director, Department of Thoracic Medicine and Honorary Consultant, Royal Brompton National Heart and Lung Hospital, London

## Kian Fan Chung MD FRCP
Senior Lecturer and Honorary Consultant Physician in Thoracic Medicine, National Heart and Lung Institute and Royal Brompton National Heart and Lung Hospital, London

## Timothy W. Evans BSc MD FRCP PhD
Reader in Critical Care, National Heart and Lung Institute; Consultant in Thoracic Medicine and Intensive Care, Royal Brompton National Heart and Lung Hospital; Consultant Physician, Westminster Hospital, London

## Stephen G. Spiro BSc MD FRCP
Consultant Physician and Honorary Senior Lecturer, Royal Brompton National Heart and Lung Hospital, University College Hospital and Middlesex Hospital, London

with a contribution by

## Robert F. Miller MB BS MRCP
Senior Lecturer in Medicine, University College London Medical School, Middlesex Hospital, London

CHURCHILL LIVINGSTONE
EDINBURGH LONDON MADRID MELBOURE NEW YORK AND TOKYO 1994

CHURCHILL LIVINGSTONE
Medical Division of Longman Group UK Limited

Distributed in the United States of America by
Churchill Livingstone Inc., 650 Avenue of the Americas,
New York, N.Y. 10011, and by associated companies,
branches and representatives throughout the world.

First published 1994

ISBN 0-443-04134-2

**British Library Cataloguing in Publication Data**
A catalogue record for this book is available from the
British Library.

**Library of Congress Cataloging in Publication Data**
Therapeutics in respiratory disease / Peter J. Barnes ... (et al.),
   with contribution by Robert F. Miller.
      p. cm.
   Includes index.
   ISBN 0-443-04134-2
   1. Lungs--Diseases--Chemotherapy.
   2. Respiratory agents.
   I. Barnes, Peter J., 1946-,
(DNLM: 1. Lung Diseases--drug therapy. WF 600 T398
1994)
RC735. C47T48 1994
616.2'00461--dc20
DNLM/DLC
for Library of Congress

Produced by Longman Singapore Publishers Pte. Ltd.
Printed in Singapore

# Preface

In recent times there have been major changes in the use and type of drugs to treat respiratory diseases. This has evolved from the introduction of many new classes of drugs, but has also arisen from a better understanding of the disease processes involved. In no disease is this more striking than in asthma, where inhaled steroids have moved from a medication that used to be added when control was not achieved with bronchodilators, to their use as first-line therapy for most patients. Advances in other respiratory diseases are also apparent. This book describes the drug treatments currently available for the management of lung diseases, and also gives some consideration to new treatments under development. We have concentrated on the drugs themselves, including their mode of action, side effects and how they should best be used. We have not set out to write a textbook of respiratory medicine as many excellent comprehensive books are already available, but have specifically considered the drugs used to treat respiratory conditions in a depth which is not provided by these books, even though this is often the most important information needed in the management of the respiratory patient.

When we agreed to put this book together we thought it important to write an integrated text, and to avoid the multiauthor format adopted by most modern textbooks. This was made easier by the fact that we work together in the same hospital and share a common treatment approach.

In putting together this book we would like to thank Churchill Livingstone for their invaluable help and advice, and also our secretaries Madeleine Wray, Patricia Lenihan and Janis House, who have all contributed enormously. We also thank Dr Norman Horne for his valuable advice and contribution on the chapter dealing with tuberculosis therapy. We hope that the book will prove to be of value to all respiratory physicians, to clinical pharmacologists and to researchers interested in lung diseases.

London 1994

P.J.B.
K.F.C.
T.W.E.
S.G.S.

# Contents

Preface  vii

**1.** General principles  1

**2.** Obstructive airway diseases  13

**3.** Respiratory failure  49

**4.** Respiratory infections  67

**5.** Opportunistic infections in the acquired immune deficiency syndrome  85

**6.** Tuberculosis  97

**7.** Lung cancer  115

**8.** Pulmonary vascular disease  131

**9.** Treatment of cough and breathlessness  153

**10.** Drug-induced pulmonary disease  161

Index  167

CHAPTER CONTENTS

**Pharmacokinetics   1**
Absorption   1
Distribution   2
Clearance   2

**Pharmacodynamics   3**
Receptors   3
Second messengers   4
   G-proteins   4
   G-protein coupled receptors   5
   Tyrosine kinase receptors   6
   Ion channel receptors   6
   Receptors regulating gene transcription   6
Drug–Receptor interaction   7

**Enzymes   8**

**Routes of delivery   9**
Inhaled route   9
   Particle size   9
   Pharmacokinetics   9
   Delivery methods   9
      Metered dose inhalers   9
      Spacer chambers   10
      Dry powder inhalers   10
      Nebulisers
Oral route   10
Parenteral therapy   11

**1**

# General principles

This first chapter describes some of the general principles involved in the drug therapy of respiratory diseases. Many factors are involved in the delivery of a drug to its site of action and are considered under *pharmacokinetics*, whereas *pharmacodynamics* involves the mechanism of action of the drug, including its interaction with receptors or enzymes and the secondary events which lead to the typical tissue response.

## PHARMACOKINETICS

In order to produce the intended pharmacological response it is necessary to achieve an effective concentration of a drug at its site of action in the lung. Several steps are involved in determining the concentration of a drug at its site of action; these include *absorption*, *distribution* to various tissues, *metabolism* and finally *excretion* (Box 1.1).

## Absorption

Absorption of drugs involves their passage across a cell membrane. For some drugs this may involve specially mediated transport systems or movement through specific channels, but for most drugs this involves simple diffusion down a concentration gradient. The rate of transport depends on the lipid solubility of the drug. Most drugs exist in solution as weak acids or weak bases and there is therefore an equilibrium between the ionised form which does not

---

**Box 1.1    Factors determining drug concentration at site of action**

Absorption
Distribution
Metabolism
Clearance
Excretion

---

readily penetrate lipid membranes and the non-ionised fraction which is lipophilic and may cross the cell membrane. The equilibrium between ionised and non-ionised forms is determined by the pKa of the drug, which is defined as the pH at which 50% of the drug is in the ionised state. As an example, sodium cromoglycate is a weak acid with a pKa of 2. At physiological pH it exists almost entirely in an ionised state and is therefore not absorbed from the gastrointestinal tract, which is why it must be delivered directly to the lungs.

Lipid solubility is also important in determining whether absorbed drugs may cross the blood–brain barrier and exert central effects. Highly lipophilic compounds such as ethanol and nicotine readily cross the blood–brain barrier. Atropine also crosses the blood–brain barrier which results in central nervous system side-effects such as hallucinations, but its quaternary derivative ipratropium bromide is ionised and has low lipid solubility, so that it is not able to cross the blood–brain barrier and central side-effects, which limit the use of atropine, are not seen. Similarly the non-sedative antihistamine cetirizine differs from its parent drug hydroxizine by the presence of a carboxyl group which makes the drug less lipophilic so that central side-effects such as sedation are avoided.

## Distribution

The concentration of a drug which is obtained at the site of action is determined by the volume of distribution of the drug, its clearance and the half-life of the drug. The volume of distribution ($V_d$) describes the body space available to con-

tain the drug. Thus for parenteral drugs which are extensively bound to plasma proteins the volume of distribution will be largely confined to the vascular space, whereas for drugs which are lipid soluble the volume of distribution will be much greater as the drug is taken up into adipose tissues throughout the body. The concentration of a drug in the blood (C) is determined by the equation:

$$C = \text{Drug dose}/V_d$$

For example, the $V_d$ for theophylline is approximately 35 l in a 70 kg person. An approximate loading dose required to give a 'therapeutic' plasma concentration of 15 mg/l would therefore be C x $V_d$ or 15 mg/l x 35 l = 525 mg. If $V_d$ is reduced by disease such cardiac or renal failure, then a correspondingly lower dose is necessary to give the same plasma concentration and to avoid toxic doses.

## Clearance

The clearance of a drug describes its elimination from biological fluids; the half-life ($t_{\frac{1}{2}}$) is the time required to eliminate 50% of a drug from the body, after absorption and distribution are complete. Although clearance and half-life may readily be established for systemically administered drugs, little is known about the clearance of inhaled drugs since the local concentrations in the lungs are not known.

Systemically administered drugs are biotransformed to an inactive state which usually involves oxidation, reduction or hydrolysis, converting the drug to more polar forms that may be more readily excreted by the kidney. Biotransformation usually takes place in the liver, but for inhaled drugs biotransformation may also take place in the lungs. Hepatic metabolism of drugs may be increased if metabolising enzymes are induced by drugs such as phenobarbitone and rifampicin, which increase the activity of cytochrome P450 related oxidative enzymes. This results in more rapid elimination of theophylline and will require an increased dose of theophylline to maintain therapeutic levels. Conversely other drugs such as cimetidine, erythromycin and ciprofloxacin may inhibit P450 associated enzymes and may lead to toxic levels of theophylline.

Excretion of drugs may be via several routes. The kidneys are the most important organs of excretion and drugs are filtered in the glomerular filtrate, although some reabsorption in the renal tubules may occur. Hydrophilic drugs are not reabsorbed, but lipophilic drugs may be reabsorbed and therefore have a longer plasma half-life. Some organic acids and bases are also actively secreted into the urine by tubular cells. The liver may also excrete drugs into the bile. The lung is an important excretory organ for gaseous and volatile substances. Lipophilic agents such as ether are rapidly excreted by this route.

## PHARMACODYNAMICS

Pharmacodynamics describes the interactions between drugs and target cells which result in a response. Two major targets for drug action are interactions with receptors and with enzymes.

## Receptors

Receptors are proteins which are usually expressed at the cell membrane that serve as specific recognition sites for extracellular stimuli. The genes for many receptors have now been cloned, which has made it possible to elucidate their amino acid sequence and tertiary structure. It has become clear that many receptors belong to large 'supergene families' with common structural features (Box 1.2). Thus receptors, such as $\beta$-adrenergic and muscarinic receptors, which interact with coupling guanine nucleotide regulatory proteins (G-proteins) all share a common structure characterised by seven transmembrane spanning elements, with extracellular components which are often glycosylated and intracellular loops which interact with the G-protein (Fig. 1.1). Binding of the agonist or antagonist appears to occur in a deep binding cleft between particular transmembrane segments. By contrast the receptors for most cytokines and growth factors comprise a long amino acid chain which crosses the cell membrane only once with large extracellular portions that interact with the protein agonist.

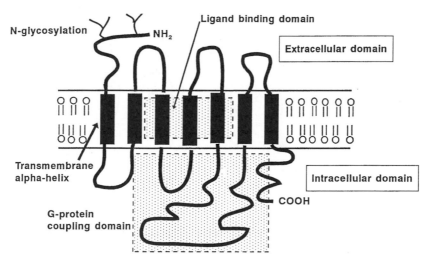

**Fig. 1.1** The general structure of a G-protein coupled receptor with seven transmembrane spanning segments. Each hydrophobic membrane spanning segment is in the form of an $\alpha$-helix. Extracellular loops may be glycosylated and intracellular loops (particularly the large third intracellular loop) interact with G-proteins. The ligand binding site is often deep within the membrane between the membrane spanning segments.

**Box 1.2    G-protein coupled receptors: some examples**

$\beta$-adrenoceptors ($\beta_1$, $\beta_2$, $\beta_3$)
$\alpha$-adrenoceptors ($\alpha_1$, $\alpha_2$)
Dopamine receptors ($D_1$, $D_2$, $D_3$)
Muscarinic cholinergic receptors ($M_1$, $M_2$, $M_3$, $M_4$)
Tachykinin receptors ($NK_1$, $NK_2$, $NK_3$)
Adenosine receptors ($A_1$, $A_2$)
Histamine receptors ($H_1$, $H_2$, $H_3$)
Leukotriene receptors ($LTB_4$, $LTD_4$)
Platelet-activating factor receptors
Thromboxane receptors

While most receptors are expressed on the cell surface, some receptors such as glucocorticosteroid receptors are intracellular and interact with DNA in the cell nucleus to alter the rate of transcription of certain genes.

It is possible to study the interaction of drugs and receptors directly using the technique of radioligand binding, using a labelled agonist or, more usually, a labelled antagonist. For example $\beta$-receptors are often characterised using the potent labelled antagonist [$^{125}$I]iodocyanopin-dolol. With this technique it is possible to study the number of binding sites (receptors) in a particular tissue, and also to determine the affinity of binding of agonists and antagonists to the same binding sites.

## Second messengers

Binding of an agonist to its receptor initiates a chain of events which eventually leads to a tissue response. While there are many different types of receptor on the cell surface, there are few intracellular mechanisms for transducing this interaction (second messengers) (Box 1.3). Thus receptors are the main determinant of tissue responsiveness.

### G-proteins

Most receptors are linked to second messenger systems via G-proteins and recently several distinct types of G-protein have been characterised pharmacologically and with the use of specific toxins and several types of G-protein have been

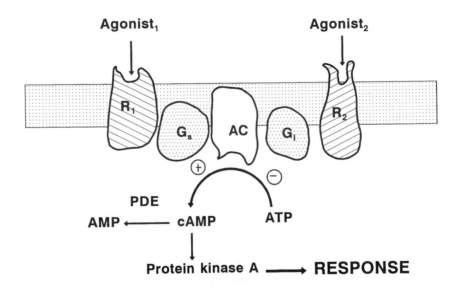

**Fig. 1.2**    Some receptors ($R_1$–e.g. ß-receptors) may stimulate adenylyl cyclase (AC) via a stimulatory G-protein ($G_s$), resulting in increased formation of cyclic 3'5' adenosine monophosphate (cAMP), the second messenger. Other receptors ($R_2$ –e.g. $M_2$ muscarinic receptors) inhibit AC via an inhibitory G-protein ($G_i$). cAMP is broken down by phosphodiesterases (PDE) to inactive AMP.

from the receptor to the effector mechanism. The $\beta$ and $\gamma$ subunits are relatively inert and stabilise the $\alpha$-subunit, acting as an anchor in the cell membrane.

### G-protein coupled receptors

Some receptors, such as $\beta_2$-adrenoceptors, are coupled to a G-protein which has a stimulatory $\alpha$-subunit ($G_s$) which stimulates the cell-associated enzyme *adenylyl cyclase* resulting in an increase in intracellular cyclic 3'5' adenosine monophosphate (cAMP) concentration. Cyclic AMP (the second messenger) then leads to activation of protein kinase A, which phosphorylates certain proteins leading to the characteristic cellular response such as relaxation of airway smooth muscle cells (Fig. 1.2).

Other receptors (e.g. muscarinic $M_2$ receptors) are linked to adenylyl cyclase via an *inhibitory* G-protein ($G_i$), which inhibits the enzyme, resulting in a fall in intracellular cyclic AMP,

cloned. G-proteins consist of three subunits; the $\alpha$-subunit interacts with both the receptor and the effector mechanism (enzyme or ion channel) and acts as a shuttle transferring information

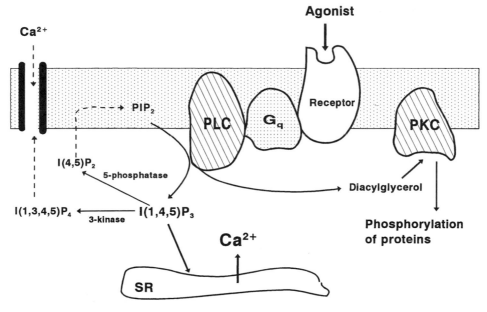

**Fig. 1.3**   Some receptors (R) lead to phosphoinositide hydrolysis via a G-protein ($G_q$) which stimulates phospholipase C (PLC). PLC converts phosphoinositide (4,5)bisphosphate ($PIP_2$) to inositol (1,4,5)trisphosphate ($IP_3$) which releases calcium ions ($Ca^{2+}$) from intracellular stores (sarcoplasmic reticulum: SR). $IP_3$ is then metabolised back to inositol which is re-incorporated into the cell membrane. $PIP_2$ also forms diacylglycerol which activates protein kinase C (PKC), which may mediate more chronic effects of receptor stimulation.

and thus opposes the effects of agonists which stimulate the enzyme.

Yet other receptors produce cellular effects by releasing *calcium ions* ($Ca^{2+}$) from intracellular stores. This occurs by the coupling of receptors via specific G-proteins (including $G_i$ and $G_q$) to the enzyme phospholipase C (or phosphoinositidase C), which breaks down the phospholipid phosphoinositide (4,5)bisphosphate to inositol (1,4,5)trisphosphate ($IP_3$), which binds to intracellular stores of calcium leading to $Ca^{2+}$ release (Fig. 1.3). Many of the mediators which contract airway smooth muscle (such as histamine, leukotrienes and acetylcholine) do so via activation of phosphoinositide hydrolysis, and inhibition of this mechanism may be an important site of action of bronchodilator drugs.

### Tyrosine kinase receptors

Another second messenger system which has not been investigated in detail in lung cells involves *tyrosine kinase*, which is an integral part of the receptor structure (Fig. 1.4). These receptors include receptors for epithelial growth factor and insulin. Tyrosine kinase phosphorylates tyrosine residues on proteins which in some

way alter the transcription of certain genes, leading to proliferative responses. The identity of these proteins is not yet certain, but several growth factor receptors, associated with cell proliferation, have tyrosine kinase activity.

### Ion channel receptors

Some receptors are not coupled to intracellular mechanisms but directly (usually via a G-protein) open or close ion channels in the cell membrane. The best example of this is the nicotinic cholinergic receptor which itself constitutes an ion channel, so that its activation leads directly to depolarisation of the cell. Molecular cloning has revealed that these receptors consist of several subunits which are arranged around a central aqueous pore which serves as the ion channel. This type of receptor is termed a *fast* receptor since it produces rapid cell responses due to immediate effects on ion movements (Fig. 1.5), in contrast to *slow* receptors such as the G-protein coupled receptors which involve a series of enzymatic steps before a response occurs. Fast receptors usually mediate synaptic transmission and include gamma-amino butyric acid and glutamate receptors.

### Receptors regulating gene transcription

Intracellular receptors, such as the glucocorticosteroid receptor, interact with the upstream regulatory sequence of certain genes, leading to either an increase or decrease in transcription rate and therefore rate of formation of mes senger RNA. This determines the amount of protein produced by the particular gene. For example steroids bind to intracellular glucocorticoid receptors which translocate to the cell nucleus and bind to specific sequences of nucleotides in the DNA double helix (Fig. 1.6). The DNA binding domain of the steroid receptor contains two loops called *zinc fingers* which are believed to wrap around the DNA double helix. This activates or inhibits transcription of steroid-sensitive target genes. For example, steroids increase transcription of the $\beta_2$-receptor

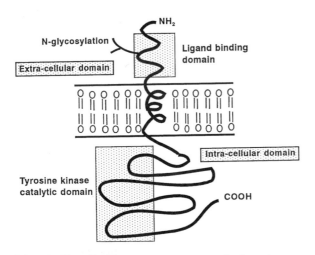

**Fig. 1.4** Tyrosine kinase receptors are a single amino acid chain with large intracellular and extracellular domains. The extracellular domain interacts with the ligand, whereas the intracellular domain has intrinsic tyrosine kinase activity.

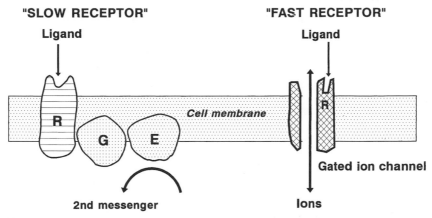

**Fig. 1.5**  G-protein coupled receptors are known as 'slow' receptors because producing a response involves a series of enzyme mediated effects. Other receptors (such as the nicotinic cholinergic receptor) are known as 'fast' receptors since they incorporate an ion channel which opens very rapidly in response to agonist activation.

gene leading to increased expression of $\beta_2$-receptors at the cell surface, whereas they inhibit the gene coding for many cytokines, including interleukin-1.

Many cytokines themselves produce their effects by regulating the transcription of particular target genes. The precise steps in this pathway are usually unknown, but involve the activation of specific protein *transcription* factors in the cytoplasm.

## Drug–Receptor interaction

The binding of a drug to its receptor is a dynamic process and follows the laws of mass action. At equilibrium there is a balance between the rate of association and the rate of dissociation of a drug. The *affinity* of the drug describes the balance between association and dissociation and can be quantified as the dissociation constant $K_d$, which is the logarithm of the concentration of drug needed to occupy 50% of the receptors. Drugs with a low $K_d$ therefore have a high affinity for their receptor.

After binding to the receptor the response is activated via second messenger systems described above. Different agonists may elicit variable degrees of response, which is described as *efficacy*. A drug that produces less than a

maximal response is known as a *partial agonist*. In airway smooth muscle isoprenaline is a full agonist and produces a maximal response, whereas salbutamol acts as a partial agonist, giving less than the maximal relaxation seen with isoprenaline. Antagonists have zero efficacy.

Antagonists block the effects of an agonist by interfering with its binding to the receptor. When antagonists interact with agonists at a common receptor the antagonism is competitive. This can be demonstrated by a rightward shift in the log concentration–response curve (Fig. 1.7). For true competitive antagonism (e.g. between a $\beta_2$-antagonist and $\beta$-agonist in airway smooth muscle) the shift is parallel. The amount of shift observed with each concentration of agonist can be used to calculate the affinity of the antagonist for the particular receptor. Sometimes a drug interferes with an agonist effect in a non-competitive manner by inhibiting any of the steps which lead to the typical agonist effect. This results in a non-parallel shift in the agonist dose–response curve and a reduced maximal response.

Another type of antagonism which is relevant to lung diseases is *functional antagonism* which describes an interaction between two agents which have opposite functional effects on the same cell system. Thus $\beta$-agonists act as func-

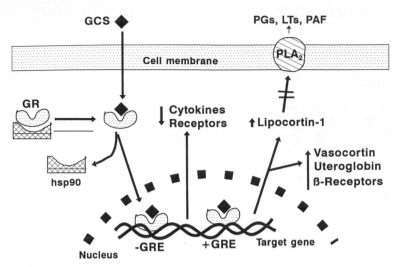

**Fig. 1.6** Glucocorticosteroid receptors (GR) interact with steroids in the cytoplasm and then translocate to the nucleus where they interact with glucocorticoid responsive elements (GRE) which either increase (+GRE) or decrease (-GRE) the rate of gene transcription.

tional antagonists in airway smooth muscle since they counteract the contractile effects of any spasmogen, including histamine, leukotriene $D_4$, thromboxane, bradykinin and acetylcholine.

Two drugs may interact to produce effects which are more than additive. If two drugs given together produce an effect which is greater than the additive effect of the drugs given separately this is known as *synergism*. *Potentiation* is when one drug given alone has no effect, but increases the response to a second drug. *Tolerance* refers to a diminishing response to a drug which is administered repeatedly, whereas *tachyphylaxis* usually describes tolerance of rapid onset, so that it may be seen after only one administration of the drug. *Desensitisation* is a term which includes rapid and long-term loss of response.

## ENZYMES

Many drugs produce their therapeutic effect by inhibition of particular enzymes. Most commonly the drug molecule is a substrate analogue which acts as a *competitive inhibitor*. The interaction between drug and enzyme obeys the law of mass action and may be analysed in the same way as drug–receptor interactions. An example is L-N$^G$-nitro arginine which acts as a competitive inhibitor of nitric oxide synthase (which generates nitric oxide in endothelial cells) by substituting for the natural substrate L-arginine. The enzyme blockade may be overcome by increasing the concentration of L-arginine. D-arginine which is not a substrate for this

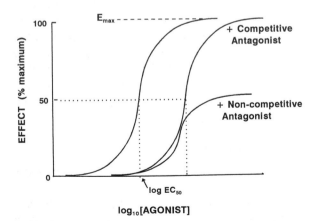

**Fig. 1.7** Concentration–response curve for drug–receptor interactions. With a competitive antagonist there is a parallel rightward shift of the curve, whereas with a non-competitive antagonist the maximum response is also reduced.

enzyme has no effect, however. Many drugs act non-competitively. An example is aspirin which non-competitively blocks cyclo-oxygenase by acetylating the active (catalytic) site of the enzyme. Another type of interaction involves a false substrate, where the drug undergoes chemical transformation by the enzyme to form a product which subverts the normal metabolic pathway. The best example of this is $\alpha$-methyldopa which mimics deoxyphenylalanine (DOPA), causing noradrenaline to be replaced by methylnoradrenaline, which is inactive.

Enzymes are increasingly recognised as playing an important part in the pathophysiology of various diseases and may become an increasingly important target for drug therapy in the future. Drugs which inhibit 5-lipoxygenase, which generates leukotrienes, have now been developed and are being tested in asthma. Drugs which inhibit neutrophil elastase may be useful in the management of cystic fibrosis and emphysema, whereas drugs which inhibit tryptase and chymase from mast cells may be useful as anti-inflammatory treatments in asthma.

## ROUTES OF DELIVERY

Drugs may be delivered to the lungs by oral or parenteral routes, but also by inhalation. The choice depends on the drug and on the respiratory disease.

## Inhaled route

Inhalation is the preferred mode of delivery of many drugs with a direct effect on airways, particularly for asthma and chronic obstructive airways disease (COAD). It is the only way to deliver some drugs such as sodium cromoglycate and anticholinergics and is the preferred route of delivery for $\beta$-agonists and corticosteroids. Antibiotics may also be delivered by inhalation in patients with chronic respiratory sepsis (e.g. in cystic fibrosis). The major advantage of inhalation is the delivery of drugs to the airways in doses which are effective with a much lower risk of side-effects. This is particularly important with the use of inhaled corticosteroids. In addition, drugs such as bronchodilators have a more rapid onset of action than when taken orally so that more rapid control of symptoms is possible.

### Particle size

The size of particles for inhalation is of critical importance in determining the site of deposition in the respiratory tract. The optimum size for particles to settle in the airways is 2–5 $\mu$m but for parenchymal deposition (needed for nebulised pentamidine in the prophylaxis of *Pneumocystis carinii* in patients with human immunodeficiency virus (HIV) infection) particle sizes of 1–2 $\mu$m may be optimal. Larger particles settle out in the upper airways, whereas smaller particles remain suspended and are therefore exhaled.

### Pharmacokinetics

Of the total drug delivered probably less than 5% enters the lower airways. The fate of the inhaled drug is poorly understood. Drugs are absorbed from the airway lumen and have direct effects on target cells of the airway. Drugs may also be absorbed into the bronchial circulation and distributed to more peripheral airways. Whether drugs are metabolised in the airways is often uncertain and there is little understanding of the factors that may influence local absorption and metabolism of inhaled drugs. Nevertheless, it is known that several drugs have great therapeutic efficacy when given by the inhaled route.

### Delivery methods

Several ways of delivering inhaled drugs are possible:

*Metered dose inhalers* (MDI). Drugs are propelled from a canister with a freon propellant (although alternative 'ozone friendly' propellants are now under development). These devices are convenient, portable and deliver

100–200 doses of drug. They are usually easy to use for adults, although it is necessary to give careful instructions. The patient must co-ordinate inhalation with action of the device, so it is important that patients are taught to use these devices correctly. These devices are unsuitable for young children.

*Spacer chambers.* There are several advantages of using large volume spacers (Box 1.4). Large volume spacer devices (e.g. Volumatic[R] or Nebuhaler[R]) between the MDI and the patient reduce the velocity of particles entering the upper airways and the size of the particles by allowing evaporation of liquid propellant. This reduces the amount of drug which impinges on the oropharynx and increases the proportion of drug entering the lower airways. The need for careful co-ordination between activation and inhalation is also avoided, since the MDI can be activated into the chamber and the aerosol subsequently inhaled from the one-way valve. Perhaps the most useful application of spacer chambers is in the reduction of the oropharyngeal deposition of inhaled steroids and thus the local side-effects of these drugs. Large volume spacers also reduce the systemic side-effects of drugs, since less drug is deposited in the oropharynx and therefore swallowed; it is the swallowed fraction of the drug, absorbed from the gastrointestinal tract, which makes the greatest contribution to the systemic fraction. This again is of particular importance in the use of inhaled steroids. Spacer devices are also useful in delivering inhaled drugs to small children who are not able to use an MDI. Children as young as 3 years are able to use a spacer device fitted with a face mask.

*Dry powder inhalers.* Drugs may also be delivered as a dry powder using devices which scatter a fine powder dispersed by air turbulence on inhalation. These devices may be preferred by some patients, since careful co-ordination is not as necessary as with the MDI, but some patients find the dry powder is irritant. Multiple dose dry powder inhalers are now available, which are more convenient. One such device, the Turbohaler, delivers 50–200

---

**Box 1.4  Advantages of large volume spacer devices**

- Less co-ordination needed for efficient inhalation

- Increased delivery to peripheral airways

- Less deposition in oropharynx
  reduced local effects
  reduced systemic absorption

- Relatively large doses of MDIs may be administered

---

doses of pure drug and therefore avoids the problems of additives such as surfactants which are necessary in MDIs and which may provoke throat irritation, coughing and even a fall in lung function in sensitive asthmatic patients. Dry powder inhalers are also easier to use in children.

*Nebulisers.* Two types of nebuliser are available. Jet nebulisers are driven by a stream of gas (air or oxygen), whereas ultrasonic nebulisers utilise a rapidly vibrating piezo-electric crystal and thus do not require a source of compressed gas. The nebulised drug may be inspired during tidal breathing and it is possible to deliver much higher doses of drug. Nebulisers are therefore useful in treating acute exacerbations of asthma, for delivering drugs when airway obstruction is extreme (e.g. in severe COAD), for delivering inhaled drugs to infants and small children who cannot use the other inhalational devices, and for delivering drugs such as antibiotics when relatively high doses must be delivered.

## Oral route

Drugs for treatment of pulmonary diseases may also be given orally. The oral dose is much higher than the inhaled dose required to achieve the same effect (by a ratio of more than 20:1), so that systemic side-effects are far more common. When there is a choice of inhaled or oral route for a drug (e.g. $\beta$-agonist or corticosteroid) the inhaled route is always preferable and the oral route should be reserved for the few patients unable to use inhalers (e.g. small children, patients with physical problems such as severe arthritis of the hand). Theophylline is ineffective by the inhaled route and therefore must be given orally. Corticosteroids may have to be given orally for parenchymal lung diseases (e.g. in interstitial lung diseases), although it may be possible in the future to deliver such drugs into alveoli using specially designed inhalational devices.

## Parenteral therapy

The intravenous route should be reserved for delivery of drugs in the severely ill patient who is unable to absorb drugs from the gastrointestinal tract. Side effects are generally frequently due to the high plasma concentrations.

FURTHER READING

Barnes P J 1988 General pharmacologic principles. In: Murray J F, Nadel J A(eds) Textbook of respiratory medicine. W B Saunders, Philadelphia, p 221–248
Barnes P J 1989 Airway receptors. Postgraduate Medical Journal 65: 532–542
Barnes P J 1990 Molecular biology of receptors: implications for lung disease. Thorax 45: 482–488
Barnes P J 1992 Pulmonary pharmacology. In: Melmon K L,

Morelli H F, Hoffman B B, Nierenberg D W (eds) Clinical pharmacology, 3rd edn. McGraw Hill, New York, p 186–218
Goodman A G, Goodman L S, Gilman A (eds) 1990 The pharmacological basis of therapeutics. MacMillan, New York.
Newman SP 1992 Delivery systems. In: Drugs for asthma, 2nd edn. IBC Publications, London, p 245–257

CHAPTER CONTENTS

**Introduction  13**
Definitions  13
Epidemiology  14
Pathophysiology  14

**Bronchodilators  16**
ß-adrenergic agonists  16
Anticholinergics  23
Theophylline  26

**Anti-inflammatory agents  30**
Corticosteroids  30
Sodium cromoglycate  36
Other anti-allergic drugs  37
Immunosuppressive therapy  38

**Clinical application  38**
Asthma  38
COAD  42

**Drugs contraindicated in airway disease  44**
Sedatives  44
ß-blockers  44
Aspirin  45
ACE inhibitors  45

**New drugs  45**
Long-acting inhaled ß$_2$-agonists  45
Potassium channel activators  45
Selective phosphodiesterase inhibitors  46
Mediator antagonists/inhibitors  46
Immunomodulators  46

# 2

# Obstructive airway diseases

## INTRODUCTION

## Definitions

### Asthma

Asthma is recognised as airway obstruction which reverses spontaneously or with therapy, and is characterised clinically by varying severity of wheeze, dyspnoea and cough. Although most asthma is easy to recognise, clinically there may be problems in older patients when airflow obstruction may become less reversible. At a pathological level asthma is characterised by a *chronic desquamative eosinophilic bronchitis*.

### Chronic obstructive airways disease (COAD)

COAD (also known as chronic obstructive pulmonary disease or chronic airflow limitation) is airways obstruction which is not reversible, and is usually related to cigarette smoking. COAD is due to *emphysema* (destruction of lung parenchyma) or to obstruction of small airways. However, patients with asthma may also have COAD. The definition of COAD is overly pessimistic since, although there is not the same reversibility which occurs in asthma, significant clinical improvement is possible in many patients with bronchodilators. Pharmacologically a major distinction between asthma and COAD is the response to steroids. Most asthmatic patients will improve (many markedly) with corticosteroids, whereas any improvement in COAD is marginal and a significant improvement in airflow obstruction would suggest a diagnosis of asthma.

### Chronic bronchitis

Chronic bronchitis implies mucus hypersecretion and is not associated with airflow obstruction. This is usually associated with smoking and resolves when smoking is stopped.

## Epidemiology

### Asthma

Asthma has now become the commonest chronic disease in industrialised countries with a cumulative prevalence as high as 25% in some countries. Numerous epidemiological studies have recently been performed to document the prevalence of asthma in different countries. Epidemiological studies have been beset with difficulties because of differing definitions of asthma and the variable nature of asthma symptoms. Most authorities now agree, however, that the prevalence of asthma has increased over the last 20 years, even taking into account differences in diagnostic fashions. These trends are seen in both developed and developing countries. The epidemiological surveys have also highlighted the fact that asthma remains underdiagnosed and only half the children with asthma are diagnosed and therefore receive appropriate therapy. There is also evidence that more patients now consult their general practitioner with asthma, and more patients are being admitted to hospital with acute asthma attacks. The statistic that has attracted most attention is the increase in asthma mortality which has occurred in several countries over the last decade. This was most marked in New Zealand. In a few countries (New Zealand and the UK) asthma mortality is now falling again, but in most countries mortality is continuing to rise. The fact that mortality from asthma is not declining goes against the trend for all other common treatable conditions.

The therapy for asthma has also increased over the last 10 years, although many patients with asthma remain untreated, are undertreated or treated with inappropriate therapies. The striking finding in all surveys of asthma deaths has been undertreatment with steroids. Indeed, anti-inflammatory therapies count for only a small proportion (less than 20%) of total treatments prescribed for asthma in many countries, despite the fact that asthma is an inflammatory condition. The most recent prescribing figures for the UK indicate that there has been some increase in the proportion of prescriptions for anti-inflammatory therapy, possibly as a result of increased awareness of asthma by general practitioners.

### COAD

Epidemiological studies have also been difficult in COAD in view of the problems of diagnosis in the community. COAD is associated with long-term smoking and its incidence is relatively high in countries with high cigarette consumption. The risk of death from COAD is some 30 times greater from heavy smokers (over 25 cigarettes/day) than from non-smokers. Smoking accounts for 80-90% of cases of COAD. Certain evidence of emphysema can only be obtained at post-mortem examination but, in a series of more than 1800 autopsies, severe emphysema was absent in non-smokers and present in up to 19% of patients consuming more than 20 cigarettes daily.

## Pathophysiology

### Asthma

Our understanding of asthma has changed markedly over the last few years. Asthma is now recognised as a chronic inflammatory disease of the airways, and even the mildest of asthmatic patients have features of inflammation in the airway mucosa. While in the past treatment was dominated by bronchodilators which relieve bronchoconstriction it now seems more logical to introduce prophylactic anti-inflammatory treatment at a much earlier stage

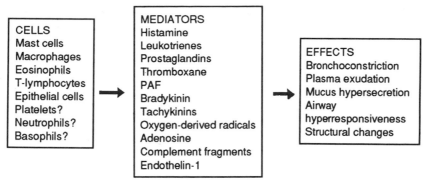

**Fig. 2.1** Inflammatory cells, mediators and effects in asthma.

in therapy. Indeed, there is little evidence that airway smooth muscle is abnormally sensitive to bronchoconstrictors in asthma, and this has focused attention on the inflammatory response in asthmatic airways which may lead to airway hyperresponsiveness.

The precise mechanisms involved in asthmatic inflammation are still debated. Several inflammatory cells appear to be involved, including mast cells, macrophages, T-lymphocytes and eosinophils (Fig. 2.1). Eosinophilic inflammation is very characteristic of asthmatic airways and indeed asthma may be considered pathologically to be chronic eosinophilic bronchitis. Several inflammatory mediators are likely to be involved, including histamine, prostaglandins, leukotrienes, platelet activating factor and bradykinin, as well as cytokines such as interleukins (IL)-3, IL-4, and IL-5. Microvascular leak and oedema of the airway wall are important components of the inflammatory response, as is mucus hypersecretion in contributing to airway narrowing and airway hyperresponsiveness. Airway nerves may also contribute via reflex bronchoconstriction and neurogenic inflammation. Activation of sensory nerve endings in the asthmatic airway may lead to the common symptoms of cough and chest tightness.

## COAD

COAD may be produced by chronic bronchitis, which involves progressive obstruction of bronchi, and by emphysema which involves parenchymal destruction with loss of elastic recoil and subsequent airway narrowing. While both are different disease processes they share the same aetiological factors, and therefore both often occur together. The pharmacological management of such patients is essentially the same. Chronic brochitis is recognised by an increase in mucus secretion as a chronic productive cough. Mucus hypersecretion, resulting from chronic irritants such as cigarette smoke, impairs mucociliary clearance which predisposes to bronchial infections. However, there is little evidence that simple chronic bronchitis leads to progressive airway obstruction and only about 20% of heavy smokers develop COAD.

Emphysema is due to destruction by enzymes of lung parenchyma, resulting in a loss of the elastic recoil which normally keeps airways open. This results in airway narrowing. The enzyme responsible for parenchymal destruction is predominantly elastase derived from neutrophils and macrophages, and which may be released by cigarette smoke. This enzyme is normally counteracted by a number of serum protease inhibitors, such as $\alpha_1$-antitrypsin and $\alpha_2$-immunoglobulin, which may be oxidised and thus inactivated by cigarette smoke. Patients with an inherited deficiency of $\alpha_1$-antitrypsin have a particularly severe form of emphysema.

Progressive airway obstruction leads to chronic hypoxia which increases pulmonary vascular pressures through hypoxic vasocon-

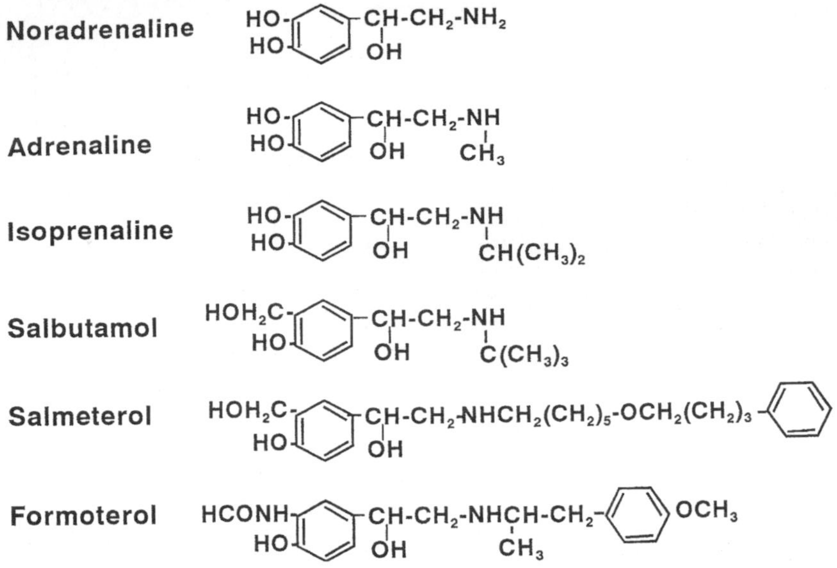

**Fig. 2.2** Chemical structure of some adrenergic agonists showing development from catecholamines.

striction and this may eventually lead to right-heart failure or cor pulmonale. In patients with emphysema destruction of the pulmonary vascular bed exacerbates this problem. Chronic hypoxaemia in some patients leads to release of erythropoietin and polycythaemia, which further exacerbates pulmonary hypertension and heart failure as blood viscosity increases.

## BRONCHODILATORS

Bronchodilator drugs have an anti-bronchoconstrictor effect, which may be demonstrated directly in vitro by a relaxant effect on precontracted airways. Bronchodilators cause immediate reversal of airway obstruction in asthma in vivo and this is believed to be due to an effect on airway smooth muscle, although additional pharmacological effects on other airway cells (such as reduced microvascular leakage and reduced release of bronchoconstrictor mediators from inflammatory cells) may contribute to the reduction in airway narrowing. Only three types of bronchodilator are in current clinical use:

*β-adrenergic agonists* (sympathomimetics)
*methylxanthines* (theophylline) and
*anticholinergic drugs.*

Drugs such as sodium cromoglycate, which prevent bronchoconstriction, have no direct bronchodilator action and are ineffective once bronchoconstriction has occurred. Corticosteroids, while gradually improving airway obstruction, have no direct effect on airway smooth muscle and are not therefore considered to be bronchodilators.

## β-adrenergic agonists

Adrenaline has been used in the treatment of asthma since the beginning of the century. Desiccated adrenal gland was originally given to asthmatic patients in the belief that it would reduce the swelling of the bronchial mucosa in the same way that it produces blanching of the skin. Adrenaline stimulates both $\alpha$- and $\beta$-adrenoceptors and, because its bronchodilator effect is mediated by $\beta$-receptors, selective $\beta$-agonists were developed. Isoprenaline, which has only $\beta$-agonist activity, was synthesised in the 1940s. Isoprenaline is a non-selective $\beta$-agonist which stimulates $\beta_1$-and $\beta_2$-receptors with equal efficacy. Because bronchodilation is mediated by $\beta_2$-receptors alone, selective $\beta_2$-agonists, such as salbutamol and terbutaline, were introduced in the 1960s.

## Chemistry

The development of $\beta_2$-agonists was a logical development of substitutions in the catecholamine structure. The catechol ring consists of hydroxyl groups in the third and fourth positions of the benzene ring (Fig. 2.2). Noradrenaline differs from adrenaline only in the terminal amine group, which therefore indicates that modification at this site confers $\beta_2$-receptor selectivity. Further substitution of the terminal amine resulted in $\beta_2$-receptor selectivity, as in salbutamol and terbutaline.

Endogenous catecholamines are rapidly removed by two active uptake processes (Fig. 2.3).

1. Uptake$_1$ is localised to sympathetic nerve terminals and noradrenaline is rapidly returned to storage vesicles.

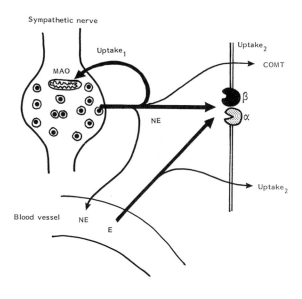

**Fig. 2.3** Uptake mechanisms for endogenous catecholamines. Noradrenaline released from adrenergic nerves is taken back up into the nerve ending by a high affinity uptake ($U_1$), where it is degraded by monoamine oxidase (MAO), whereas both noradrenaline and adrenaline are taken up by a lower affinity mechanism ($U_2$) in tissues, and subsequently degraded by catechol-o-methyl transferase (COMT).

2. Uptake$_2$ facilitates uptake into non-neuraltissue, such as smooth muscle cells, where enzymatic degradation occurs.

Isoprenaline is not a substrate for uptake$_1$, but is avidly taken up by uptake$_2$, whereas non-catecholamine $\beta$-agonists (such as salbutamol) are not taken up by either process. Catecholamines are rapidly metabolised by the enzyme catechol-o-methyl transferase (COMT), which methylates in the 3-hydroxyl position, and accounts for the short duration of action of catecholamines. Modification of the catechol ring, as in salbutamol and terbutaline, prevents this degradation and therefore prolongs their effect. Catecholamines are also broken down by monoamine oxidase (MAO) in sympathetic nerve terminals and in the gastrointestinal tract which cleaves the side chain. Isoprenaline, which is a substrate for MAO, is therefore metabolised in the gut, making absorption variable. Substitution in the amine group confers resistance to MAO and ensures reliable absorption. Many other $\beta_2$-selective agonists have now been introduced and, while there may be differences in potency, there are no clinically significant differences in selectivity. Inhaled $\beta_2$-selective drugs in current clinical use have a similar duration of action, but recently inhaled $\beta_2$-selective drugs which have a much longer duration of effect (over 12 hours), such as salmeterol and formoterol, have been developed.

## Mode of action

$\beta$-agonists produce bronchodilation by directly stimulating $\beta_2$-receptors in airway smooth muscle, which leads to relaxation. This can be

---

**Box 2.1   Mechanism of relaxation of airway smooth muscle by $\beta$-agonists**

Activation of calcium-activated potassium channels
Increased calcium ion removal pumps
Inhibition of phosphoinositide hydrolysis (which releases intracellular calcium ions)
Inhibition of myosin phosphorylation

---

**Box 2.2   Effects of β-agonists in airway cells**

Relaxation of airway smooth muscle (proximal and distal airways)
Inhibition of mast cell mediator release
Inhibition of plasma exudation and airway oedema
Increased mucociliary clearance
Increased mucus secretion
No effect on chronic inflammation

---

demonstrated in vitro by the relaxant effect of isoprenaline on human bronchi and lung strips (indicating an effect on peripheral airways), and in vivo by a rapid decrease in airway resistance. β-receptors have been demonstrated in airway smooth muscle by direct receptor binding techniques and autoradiographic studies indicate that β-receptors are localised to smooth muscle of all airways from trachea to terminal bronchioles. The molecular mechanisms by which β-agonists induce relaxation of airway smooth muscle have been extensively investigated.

Activation of adenylyl cyclase increases intracellular cyclic adenosine 3,5 monophosphate (cAMP), leading to activation of a specific kinase (protein kinase A) which causes relax-

ation by several mechanisms, including lowering of intracellular calcium ion ($Ca^{2+}$) concentration by active removal of $Ca^{2+}$ from the cell and into intracellular stores, and also by an inhibitory effect on myosin phosphorylation (Box 2.1). In addition there is the opening of a potassium channel which repolarises the smooth muscle cell and may stimulate the sequestration of $Ca^{2+}$ into intracellular stores (Fig. 2.4).

β-agonists act as *functional antagonists* and reverse bronchoconstriction irrespective of the contractile agent. This is an important property, since many bronchoconstrictor mechanisms (neural and mediators) are likely to be contributory in asthma.

β-agonists may have additional effects on airways, and β-receptors are localised to several different airway cells (Box 2.2).

- β-agonists have potent effects in preventing *mediator release* from isolated human lung mast cells both in vitro and in vivo.
- β-agonists may also reduce and prevent *microvascular leakage* and thus the development of bronchial mucosal oedema after exposure to mediators such as histamine.

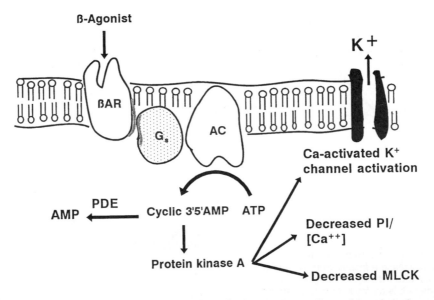

**Fig. 2.4**   Molecular mechanism of β-agonists. Activation of a $\beta_2$-receptor on the surface of an airway smooth muscle cell leads to activation of adenylyl cyclase (AC) via a coupling protein ($G_s$), leading to an increase in cyclic AMP (cAMP) concentration. cAMP is broken down by phosphodiesterases (PDE). cAMP activates protein kinase A which, in turn, activates target enzymes and ion channels as shown, leading to relaxation.

- β-agonists increase *mucus secretion* from submucosal glands and ion transport across airway epithelium; these effects may enhance mucociliary clearance, and therefore reverse the defect in clearance found in asthma.
- β-agonists may also release a *relaxant factor* (which has not yet been identified) from airway epithelial cells.
- β-agonists reduce *neurotransmission* in cholinergic nerves by an action at prejunctional $\beta_2$-receptors to inhibit acetylcholine release. This may contribute to their bronchodilator effect by reducing cholinergic reflex bronchoconstriction. In animal studies $\beta_2$-receptors on sensory nerves inhibit the release of bronchoconstrictor and inflammatory peptides such as substance P.

Although these additional effects of β-agonists may be relevant to the prophylactic use of these drugs against various challenges, their rapid bronchodilator action can probably be attributed to a direct effect on airway smooth muscle.

### Choice of drug

*Adrenaline.* Adrenaline is still the drug of choice for treatment of acute anaphylaxis, where a combination of α- and β-adrenergic agonist effects is desirable, but is now no longer the first choice for treating asthma. The disadvantages of adrenaline are its lack of β-adrenergic selectivity, resulting in $\beta_1$-receptor mediated cardiac stimulation, and its short duration of action because of rapid metabolism and

**Table 2.1   Inhaled β-agonists**

| Drug | Trade Name | Dose (µg/puff) | Comments |
|---|---|---|---|
| *Inhaled β-agonists via MDI* | | | |
| Isoprenaline | Isoprel | 100, 400 | Non-selective, short duration |
| Salbutamol | Ventolin, Aerolin, Salbulin, Salbuvent | 100 | Selective, medium duration |
| Terbutaline | Bricanyl | 250 | Selective, medium duration |
| Fenoterol | Berotec | 200 | Selective, medium duration |
| Pirbuterol | Exirel | 200 | Selective, medium duration |
| Reproterol | Bronchodil | 500 | Selective, medium duration |
| Orciprenaline | Alupent | 750 | Partially selective |
| Rimiterol | Pulmodil | 200 | Selective, short acting |
| Salmeterol | Serevent | 25 | Long-acting, use b.d. |
| *Inhaled β-agonists via dry powder inhalers* | | | |
| Salbutamol | Ventolin | 200, 400 | Rotacaps, Ventodisks |
| Terbutaline | Bricanyl | 500 | Turbohaler |
| Salmeterol | Serevent | 50 | Diskhaler |

removal by the uptake mechanisms discussed above. Its $\alpha$-agonist effects could be an advantage in reducing microvascular leakage in airways (by a vasoconstrictor effect on bronchial arterioles). Nebulised adrenaline offers no advantage over salbutamol, at least in acute severe asthma, although anecdotally some patients apparently respond better to subcutaneous adrenaline than to $\beta$-agonist aerosols. There is no convincing evidence that adrenaline causes bronchoconstriction via activation of $\alpha$-adrenergic receptors on airway smooth muscle.

*Isoprenaline.* Isoprenaline is a non-selective $\beta$-agonist and therefore may have cardiac side-effects. Pharmacologically it behaves as a full agonist, whereas $\beta_2$-selective drugs are partial agonists. Comparison of dose–response curves to isoprenaline and salbutamol, however, shows no greater bronchodilating effect with isoprenaline. Isoprenaline has a relatively short bronchodilator effect (< 2 h) because of metabolism by the enzymes COMT and MAO, although its onset is very rapid (peak effect 5 min). *Orciprenaline* is also non-selective, but is resistant to enzymatic degradation and so has a longer duration of action.

*$\beta_2$-selective agonists.* Several $\beta_2$-selective agonists are now available (Table 2.1). These drugs are as effective as non-selective agonists in their bronchodilator action, since airway effects are mediated only by $\beta_2$-receptors. However, they are less likely to produce cardiac stimulation than isoprenaline because $\beta_1$-receptors are stimulated relatively less. With the exception of rimiterol (which retains the catechol ring structure and is therefore susceptible to COMT), they have a longer duration of action because they are resistant to uptake and enzymatic degradation by COMT and MAO.

There is little to choose between the various medium-acting $\beta$-agonists currently available; all are usable by inhalation and orally, have a similar duration of action (usually 3–4 h but less in severe asthma) and similar side-effects. Differences in $\beta_2$-selectivity have been claimed but are not clinically important. Drugs in clinical use include salbutamol, terbutaline, fenoterol, rimiterol and pirbuterol. It has been claimed that fenoterol is less $\beta_2$-selective than salbutamol and terbutaline, resulting in increased cardiovascular side-effects, but this evidence is controversial, since these effects are mediated via $\beta_2$-receptors. The increased incidence of cardiovascular effects is more likely to be related to the greater effective dose of fenoterol.

*Long-acting $\beta_2$-agonists.* Inhaled $\beta_2$-agonists with a long duration of action (over 12 h) have recently been developed and have now been introduced in some countries. Formoterol and salmeterol have a bronchodilator effect of over 12 h and are therefore suitable for twice daily dosing. They are likely to be particularly useful in patients with nocturnal asthma and with unstable asthma. They should be reserved for patients with more severe asthma and who are already receiving high to moderate dose inhaled corticosteroids.

### Mode of administration

*Inhalation* is the method of choice for routine treatment, since side-effects are less likely, the therapeutic benefit may be greater and the effect is more rapid in onset. Furthermore, $\beta$-agonists may be more effective by inhalation; thus, inhaled salbutamol is able to prevent exercise-induced asthma, whereas an oral dose with similar bronchodilator effect is not. This may indicate that the inhaled drug may reach surface cells (e.g. mast cells or epithelial cells) inaccessible to the orally administered drug. $\beta$-agonists are normally given by metered dose inhaler, but several dry powder formulations are available.

*Oral* administration of $\beta$-agonists provides no advantage over the inhaled route and is more likely to be associated with side-effects. Sustained-release preparations may be useful in treating nocturnal asthma in some patients.

*Intravenous* administration is associated with more frequent side-effects and, for acute asthma, has not been shown to have any significant benefit over a nebulised $\beta$-agonist. Subcutaneous infusion of a $\beta_2$-agonist has proved useful in some asthmatic patients, with 'brittle' asthma characterised by sudden and unpredictable episodes of bronchoconstriction.

### Side-effects

Unwanted effects are dose-related and are due to stimulation of extrapulmonary $\beta$-receptors (Box 2.3). Side-effects are not common with inhaled therapy, but more common with oral or intravenous administration.

*Muscle tremor.* Muscle tremor is due to stimulation of $\beta_2$-receptors in skeletal muscle, and is the commonest side-effect. It may be more troublesome with elderly patients.

*Cardiovascular.* Tachycardia and palpitations are due to reflex cardiac stimulation secondary to peripheral vasodilation, from direct stimulation of atrial $\beta_2$-receptors (human heart is unusual in having a relatively high proportion of $\beta_2$-receptors), and possibly also from stimulation of myocardial $\beta_1$-receptors as the doses of $\beta_2$-agonist are increased. These side-effects tend to disappear with continued use of the drug, reflecting the development of tolerance.

*Metabolic.* Metabolic effects (increase in free fatty acid, insulin, glucose, pyruvate and lactate) are usually seen only after large systemic doses. *Hypokalaemia* is a potentially more serious side-effect. This is due to $\beta_2$-receptor stimulation of potassium entry into skeletal muscle, which may be secondary to a rise in insulin secretion. Hypokalaemia might be serious in the presence of hypoxia, as in acute asthma, when there may be a predisposition to cardiac dysrhythmias. In practice, significant arrhythmias after nebulised $\beta_2$-agonist have not been reported in acute asthma, however.

*Hypoxaemia.* $\beta$-agonists may increase ventilation–perfusion ($\dot{V}/\dot{Q}$) mismatching by causing pulmonary vasodilatation in blood vessels previously constricted by hypoxia, resulting in the shunting of blood to poorly ventilated areas and a fall in arterial oxygen tension. Although in practice the effect of $\beta$-agonists on $Pao_2$ is usu-ally very small (< 5mm Hg fall), occasionally in severe chronic airways obstruction it is large, although it may be prevented by giving additional inspired oxygen.

### Safety of $\beta$-agonists

Because of a possible relationship between adrenergic drug therapy and the rise in asthma deaths in the UK during the early 1960s, doubts have been cast on the safety of $\beta$-agonists. A causal relationship between $\beta$-agonist use and mortality has never been established, although in retrospective studies this would not be possible. More recently, these doubts have been revived and the use of high doses of $\beta$-agonists given by nebulisers at home was linked to the increase in asthma deaths in New Zealand. However, there is no convincing evidence that $\beta$-agonists contribute to asthma deaths, which can usually be ascribed to underestimation and under-treatment of the disease.

A particular $\beta_2$-agonist, fenoterol, has been linked to the recent rise in asthma deaths in New Zealand. However, the evidence is controversial and it is likely that any increased risk in mortality can be explained by the fact that fenoterol, as a more potent bronchodilator, was used in more severe asthmatics who are at higher risk. A recent study in Saskatchewan, Canada, examined the links between drugs dispensed for asthma and death or near death from asthma attacks, based on computerised

---

**Box 2.3  Side-effects of $\beta$-agonists**

Muscle tremor (direct effect on skeletal muscle $\beta_2$-receptors)
Tachycardia (direct effect on atrial receptors, reflex effect from increased peripheral vasodilatation via $\beta_2$-receptors)
Hypokalaemia (direct effect on skeletal muscle uptake of K+ via $\beta_2$-receptors)
Restlessness
Hypoxaemia (increased $\dot{V}/\dot{Q}$ mismatch due to pulmonary vasodilatation)
Worsening of asthma control? (controversial)

records of prescribing. There was a marked increase in the risk of death with high doses of all inhaled β-agonists. The risk was greater with fenoterol, but when the dose was adjusted to the equivalent dose for salbutamol there was no significant difference in the risk for these two drugs. The link between high β-agonist usage and increased asthma mortality does not prove a causal association, since patients with more severe and poorly controlled asthma, who are likely to have an increased risk of fatal attacks, are more likely to be using higher doses of β-agonist inhalers and also less likely to be using effective anti-inflammatory treatment. Indeed in the patients who used inhaled steroids there was a marked reduction in risk of death.

Recent evidence suggests that the regular use of inhaled β-agonists may increase asthma morbidity. In a study carried out in New Zealand the regular use of fenoterol was associated with poorer control and an increase in airway hyperirresponsiveness compared with patients using fenoterol 'on demand' for symptom control. Other studies have shown that regular inhaled β-agonists (salbutamol or terbutaline) are associated with an increase in airway responsiveness, although the magnitude of the changes described is small and of doubtful clinical significance.

It is now clear that β-agonists do not have significant anti-inflammatory effects in asthma, since unlike steroids they do not appear to suppress the chronic inflammatory process. This suggests that β-agonists should be used for symptom control and should not be given as regular therapy to control asthma symptoms, unless concomitant anti-inflammatory treatment is also prescribed. The same considerations apply to long-acting inhaled $\beta_2$-agonists and the fact that these drugs produce prolonged functional antagonism does not imply any anti-inflammatory activity.

### Tolerance

Continuous treatment with an agonist often leads to tolerance or subsensitivity, which may be due to down-regulation of the receptor. For this reason there have been many studies of bronchial β-receptor function after prolonged therapy with β-agonists. Tolerance of non-airway β-receptor responses, such as tremor and cardiovascular and metabolic responses, is readily induced in normal and asthmatic subjects. But whether tolerance of airway β-receptors occurs is debatable. Tolerance of human airway smooth muscle to β-agonists in vitro has been demonstrated, although the concentration of agonist necessary is high and the degree of desensitisation is variable. Animal studies suggest that pulmonary β-receptors may be more resistant to desensitisation than β-receptors elsewhere. In normal subjects bronchodilator tolerance has been demonstrated in some studies after high dose inhaled salbutamol, but not in others. Similarly, in asthmatic subjects tolerance has been found in some studies but not in others. However, even when tolerance has been demonstrated, the effect is very small and probably clinically insignificant; the more readily demonstrable tolerance of extrapulmonary effects has the benefit that side-effects tend to disappear with continued use. Recent evidence suggests that tolerance develops to the mast cell stabilising effect of β-agonists, but not to the bronchodilator effect; this might explain why intermittent use of β-agonists may be more effective than regular use. The reason for the relative resistance of airway smooth muscle β-receptors to desensitisation remains uncertain, but perhaps reflects the fact that, in asthmatic airways, β-receptors may always be 'down-regulated' as a result of the chronic inflammatory process.

Experimental studies have shown that corticosteroids prevent the development of tolerance in airway smooth muscle, and prevent and reverse the fall in pulmonary β-receptor density. Similarly, intravenous hydrocortisone reverses the tolerance of airway β-receptors in normal subjects. Thus, any tendency for tolerance to develop with high dose inhaled β-agonists should be prevented by concomitant administration of corticosteroids.

## Clinical use

β-agonists are the most widely used and effective bronchodilators in the treatment of asthma. When inhaled from metered dose aerosols they are convenient, easy to use, rapid in onset and without significant side-effects. In addition to an acute bronchodilator effect, they are effective in protecting against various challenges, such as exercise, cold air and allergen. They are the bronchodilators of choice in treating acute severe asthma, when the nebulised route of administration is as effective as intravenous use. The inhaled route of administration is preferable to the oral route because side-effects are less, and also because it may be more effective.

β-agonists should not be used on a regular basis in the treatment of mild asthma, but should be used as required by symptoms, since increased usage then indicates the need for more anti-inflammatory therapy.

# Anticholinergics

Datura plants, which contain the muscarinic antagonist strammonium, were smoked for relief of asthma two centuries ago. Atropine, a related naturally occurring compound, was also introduced for treating asthma but, because these compounds gave side-effects, particularly drying of secretions, less soluble quaternary compounds, such as atropine methylnitrate and ipratropium bromide, were introduced. These compounds are topically active and are not significantly absorbed from the respiratory tract.

## Mode of action

Anticholinergics are specific antagonists of muscarinic receptors and, in therapeutic use, have no other significant pharmacological effects. In animals and man there is a small degree of resting bronchomotor tone which is probably due to tonic vagal nerve impulses which release acetylcholine in the vicinity of airway smooth muscle, since it can be blocked by anticholinergic drugs (Fig. 2.5). There is considerable evidence that cholinergic pathways may

play an important role in regulating acute bronchomotor responses in animals and there are a wide variety of mechanical, chemical and immunological stimuli which are capable of eliciting reflex bronchoconstriction via vagal pathways. This suggested that cholinergic mechanisms might underlie airway hyperresponsiveness and acute bronchoconstrictor responses in asthma, with the implication that anticholinergic drugs would be effective bronchodilators in asthma. Many controlled studies have now been performed. In general, while these drugs may afford protection against acute

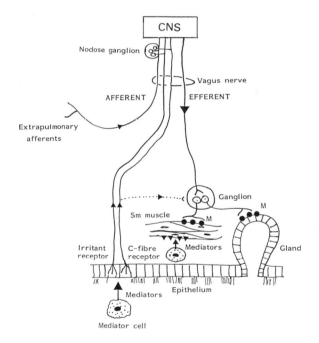

Fig. 2.5 Cholinergic neural pathways to the airways. Efferent cholinergic nerves travel in the vagus nerve and relay in ganglia situated within the airway wall, from which short postganglionic fibres travel to airway smooth muscle and glands. Anticholinergic drugs block the effects of acetylcholine released from these nerves on muscarinic receptors on the target cells. Cholinergic mechanisms may be activated via reflex mechanisms within and outside the lung. In asthma, inflammatory mediators (e.g. bradykinin) may activate sensory nerve endings in the airway to stimulate a cholinergic reflex, but other mediators (e.g. histamine and leukotrienes) act directly on airway smooth muscle cells. Thus anticholinergic drugs may not be very effective in chronic asthma compared to β-agonists which act as functional antagonists to all the mediator effects on airway smooth muscle.

challenge by sulphur dioxide, inert dusts, cold air and emotional factors, they are less effective against antigen challenge, exercise and fog. This not surprising, as anticholinergic drugs will only inhibit reflex cholinergic bronchoconstriction and could have no significant blocking effect on the direct effects of inflammatory mediators such as histamine and leukotrienes on bronchial smooth muscle. Furthermore, cholinergic antagonists probably have little or no effect on mast cells and microvascular leak.

### Ipratropium bromide

Ipratropium bromide is the most widely used anticholinergic inhaler and is available as an MDI and nebulised preparation. The onset of bronchodilation is relatively slow and is usually maximal 30–60 minutes after inhalation, but may persist for up to 8 hours. It is usually given by MDI 4 times daily on a regular basis, rather than intermittently for symptom relief, in view of its slow onset of action.

### Oxitropium bromide

Oxitropium bromide is a new quaternary anticholinergic bronchodilator which is similar to ipratropium bromide in terms of receptor blockade. It is available in higher doses by inhalation and may therefore have a more prolonged effect. Thus, it may be useful in some patients with nocturnal asthma.

### Clinical use

*Asthma.* In asthmatic subjects anticholinergic drugs are usually less effective as bronchodilators than β-agonists and offer less efficient protection against various bronchial challenges, although their duration of action is significantly longer. These drugs may be more effective in older patients with asthma. Nebulised anticholinergic drugs are effective in acute severe asthma, although they are less effective than β-agonists in this situation. Nevertheless, in the acute and chronic treatment of asthma, anticholinergic drugs may have an additive effect with β-agonists and should therefore be considered when control of asthma is not adequate with β-agonists, particularly if there are problems with theophylline, or inhaled β-agonists give troublesome tremor in elderly patients. The time course of bronchodilation with anticholinergic drugs is slower than with β-agonists, reaching a peak only 1 hour after inhalation, but persists for over 6 hours.

*COAD.* In COAD anticholinergic drugs may be as effective as, or even superior to β-agonists. Their relatively greater effect in chronic obstructive airways disease than in asthma may be explained by an inhibitory effect on vagal tone which, while not necessarily being increased in COAD, may be the only reversible element of airway obstruction which is exaggerated by geometric factors in a narrowed airway (Fig. 2.6).

### Side-effects

Inhaled anticholinergic drugs are usually well tolerated and there is no evidence for any decline in responsiveness with continued use. On stopping inhaled anticholinergics a small rebound increase in responsiveness has been described, but the clinical relevance of this is uncertain. Atropine has side-effects which are dose-related and are due to cholinergic antagonism in other systems which may lead to dryness of the mouth, blurred vision and urinary retention. Systemic side-effects after ipratropium bromide are very uncommon because there is virtually no systemic absorption (Box 2.4).

---

**Box 2.4    Side-effects of inhaled anticholinergic drugs**

Paradoxical bronchoconstriction
Glaucoma (with nebulised drug when used without mouthpiece)
Bitter taste
Systemic effects such as dry mouth: very rare

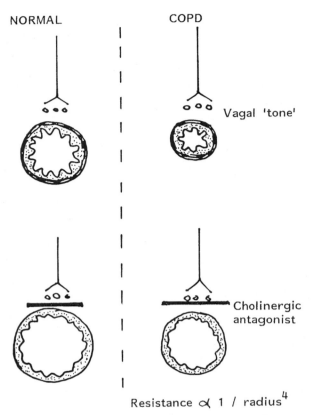

NORMAL                COPD

Vagal 'tone'

Cholinergic antagonist

Resistance $\propto$ 1 / radius$^4$

**Fig. 2.6** Anticholinergic drugs inhibit vagally mediated airway tone leading to bronchodilation. This effect is small in normal airways but is greater in airways of patients with COAD which are structurally narrowed.

*Effects on mucus secretion.* Because cholinergic agonists stimulate mucus secretion there have been several studies of mucus secretion with anticholinergic drugs as there has been concern that they may reduce secretion and lead to more viscous mucus. Atropine reduces mucociliary clearance in normal subjects and in patients with asthma and chronic bronchitis, but ipratropium bromide, even in high doses, has no detectable effect in either normal subjects or in patients with airway disease.

*Taste.* A significant unwanted effect is the unpleasant bitter taste of inhaled ipratropium, which may contribute to poor compliance with this drug.

*Glaucoma.* Nebulised ipratropium bromide may precipitate glaucoma in elderly patients due to a direct effect of the nebulised drug on the eye. This may be prevented by nebulisation with a mouthpiece rather than a face mask.

*Paradoxical bronchoconstriction.* There are several reports of paradoxical bronchoconstriction with ipratropium bromide, particularly when given by nebuliser. This is largely explained by the hypotonicity of the nebuliser solution and by antibacterial additives, such as benzalkonium chloride and ethylenediamine tetra-acetic acid (EDTA). Nebuliser solutions free of these problems are less likely to cause bronchoconstriction. Occasionally, bronchoconstriction may occur with ipratropium bromide given by MDI. It is possible that this is due to blockade of prejunctional muscarinic receptors on cholinergic nerves which normally inhibit acetylcholine release.

# Theophylline

The bronchodilator effect of strong coffee was described by Dr Hyde Salter during the last century, and methylxanthines such as theophylline, which are related to caffeine, have been used in the treatment of asthma since 1930. Indeed, theophylline is still the most widely used anti-asthma therapy world wide. Theophylline became more useful with the availability of rapid plasma assays and the introduction of reliable slow-release preparations. However, the frequency of side-effects and the relative low efficacy of theophylline have recently led to reduced usage, since β-agonists are far more effective as bronchodilators and inhaled steroids have a much greater anti-inflammatory effect. It is likely that theophylline will be less important in the future and it has now been relegated to third-line therapy. In patients with severe asthma it still remains a very useful drug, however.

## Chemistry

Theophylline is a methylxanthine similar in structure to the common dietary xanthines caffeine and theobromine. Several substituted derivatives have been synthesised but none has any advantage over theophylline, apart from the 3-propyl derivative, enprofylline, which is more potent as a bronchodilator and may have fewer toxic effects. Many salts of theophylline have also been marketed, the most common being aminophylline, which is the ethylenediamine salt used to increase solubility at neutral pH. Other salts, such as choline theophyllinate,

---

> **Box 2.5    Mode of action of theophylline**
>
> Phosphodiesterase inhibition
> Adenosine receptor antagonism
> Increased adrenaline secretion
> Prostaglandin inhibition
> Inhibition of calcium entry/release
> Inhibition of phosphoinositide hydrolysis

---

do not have any advantage and others, such as acepifylline, are virtually inactive.

## Mode of action

Although theophylline has been in clinical use for more than 50 years its mechanism of action is still uncertain. Several modes of action have been proposed (Box 2.5).

*Phosphodiesterase inhibition.* It is widely held that the bronchodilator effect of theophylline is due to inhibition of phosphodiesterase (PDE), which breaks down cyclic AMP in the cell, thereby leading to an increase in intracellular cyclic AMP concentrations. Theophylline is a non-selective PDE inhibitor, but the degree of inhibition is trivial at concentrations of theophylline which are therapeutically relevant, and there is no evidence that airway smooth muscle cells concentrate theophylline to achieve higher intracellular than circulating concentrations. Other drugs which have a greater inhibitory effect on PDE, such as dipyridamole and papaverine, have no bronchodilator effect. Furthermore, inhibition of PDE should lead to synergistic interaction with β-agonists, but this has not been convincingly demonstrated in vivo. Several isozymes of PDE have now been recognised and some are more relevant to smooth muscle relaxation. There is an indication that selective PDE inhibitors might prove useful in asthma therapy in the future. It is possible that PDE inhibition may also be relevant in mediating anti-inflammatory and immuno-modulatory roles of theophylline which may be evident at lower concentrations of theophylline than those needed for relaxation of airway smooth muscle.

*Adenosine receptor antagonism.* Theophylline is a potent inhibitor of adenosine receptors at therapeutic concentrations, suggesting that this could be the basis for its bronchodilator effects. Although adenosine has little effect on human airway smooth muscle in vitro, it causes bronchoconstriction in asthmatic subjects when given by inhalation, by releasing histamine from airway mast cells, which is prevented by therapeutic concentrations of theophylline. However, this only confirms that theophylline is capable of antagonising the effects of adenosine at therapeutic concentrations. Enprofylline, which is more potent than theophylline as a bronchodilator, has no significant inhibitory effect on adenosine receptors at therapeutic concentrations, suggesting that adenosine antagonism is an unlikely explanation for the bronchodilator effect of theophylline. However, adenosine antagonism may account for some of the side-effects of theophylline, such as central nervous system stimulation, cardiac arrhythmias and diuresis.

*Endogenous catecholamine release.* Theophylline increases the secretion of adrenaline from the adrenal medulla, although the increase in plasma concentration is small and insufficient to account for any significant bronchodilator effect.

*Prostaglandin inhibition.* Theophylline antagonises the effect of some prostaglandins or vascular smooth muscle in vitro, but there is no evidence that these effects are seen at therapeutic concentrations or are relevant to airway effects.

*Calcium influx.* There is some evidence that theophylline may interfere with calcium mobilisation in airway smooth muscle. Theophylline has no effect on entry of calcium ions ($Ca^{2+}$) via voltage-dependent channels, but it has been suggested that it may influence calcium entry via receptor-operated channels, release from intracellular stores, or have some effect on phosphatidylinositol turnover (which is linked to release of $Ca^{2+}$ from intracellular stores). There is no direct evidence in favour of this, other than an effect on intracellular cyclic AMP concentration due to its PDE inhibitory action.

*Unknown mechanisms.* Despite extensive study, it has been difficult to elucidate the molecular mechanism for the bronchodilating or other anti-asthma actions of theophylline. It is possible that any beneficial effect in asthma is related to its action on other cells (such as platelets, T-lymphocytes or macrophages) or on airway microvascular leak and oedema in addition to airway smooth muscle relaxation. Indeed theophylline is a rather ineffective bronchodilator and its anti-asthma effect is more likely to be explained by some other effect. It may be relevant that theophylline is ineffective when given by inhalation, but is effective when a critical plasma concentration is reached. This may indicate that it is having important effects on cells other than those in the airway. Theophylline may act as an immunomodulator and has effects on T-lymphocyte function, since it is apparently effective in suppressing graft rejection.

## Action of theophylline

The primary effect of theophylline is assumed to be relaxation of airway smooth muscle and in vitro studies have shown that it is equally effective in large or small airways. However, theophylline is a very weak bronchodilator at therapeutically relevant concentrations, as discussed above, suggesting that some other target cell may be more relevant. Theophylline inhibits mast cell mediator release, increases mucociliary clearance and prevents the development of microvascular leakiness and therefore has been considered 'anti-inflammatory'. Theophylline has inhibitory actions on T-lymphocytes which may be relevant to the control of chronic airway inflammation, but has no effect on eosinophil degranulation at clinically relevant concentrations, which is in agreement with its lack of effect in reducing airway hyperresponsiveness.

In addition, aminophylline apparently increases the contractility of the fatigued diaphragm in man. Whether this is relevant clinically in respiratory failure is uncertain.

## Pharmacokinetics

There is a close relationship between improvement in airway function and serum theophylline concentration. Below 10 mg/l therapeutic effects (at least in terms of rapid improvement in airway function) are small and above 25 mg/l additional benefits are outweighed by side-effects, so that the therapeutic range is usually taken as 10–20 mg/l. The dose of theophylline required to give these therapeutic concentrations varies between subjects, largely because of differences in clearance. In addition, there may be differences in bronchodilator response to theophylline and, with acute bronchoconstriction, higher concentrations may be required to produce bronchodilation.

Theophylline is rapidly and completely absorbed, but there are large inter-individual variations in clearance, due to differences in hepatic metabolism (Box 2.6). Theophylline is metabolised in the liver by the cytochrome P450/P448 microsomal enzyme system, and a large number of factors may influence hepatic metabolism.

*Increased clearance.* Increased clearance is seen in children (1–16 years), and in cigarette and marijuana smokers. Concurrent administration of phenytoin and phenobarbitone increases activity of P450, resulting in increased metabolic breakdown, so that higher doses may be required.

*Reduced clearance.* Reduced clearance is found in liver disease, pneumonia and heart failure and doses need to be reduced to half and plasma levels monitored carefully. Increased

clearance is also seen with certain drugs, including erythromycin, quinolone antibiotics (e.g. ciprofloxacin), allopurinol and cimetidine (but not ranitidine) which interfere with cytochrome P450 function. Thus, if a patient on maintenance theophylline requires a course of erythromycin, the dose of theophylline should be halved. Viral infections and vaccination may also reduce clearance, and this may be particularly important in children. Because of these variations in clearance, individualisation of theophylline dosage is required and plasma concentrations should be measured 4 h after the last dose with slow-release preparations when steady state has usually been achieved. There is no significant circadian variation in theophylline metabolism, although there may be delayed absorption at night, which may relate to the supine posture.

### Routes of administration

*Intravenous.* Intravenous aminophylline has been used for many years in the treatment of acute severe asthma. The recommended dose is now 6 mg/kg given intravenously over 20–30 min, followed by a maintenance dose of 0.5 mg/kg/h. If the patient is already taking theo phylline, or there are any factors which decrease clearance, these doses should be halved and the plasma level checked more frequently.

*Oral.* Plain theophylline tablets or elixir, which are rapidly absorbed, give wide fluctuations in plasma levels and are not recommended. Several effective sustained-release preparations are now available which are absorbed at a constant rate and provide steady plasma concentrations over a 12–24 hour period. Although there are differences between preparations, these are relatively minor and of no clinical significance. Both slow-release aminophylline and theophylline are available and are equally effective (although the ethylenediamine component of aminophylline has very occasionally been implicated in allergic reactions). For continuous treatment twice daily therapy (approximately 8 mg/kg twice daily) is

---

**Box 2.6   Factors affecting theophylline clearance**

*Increased clearance*

Enzyme induction (rifampicin, phenobarbitone, ethanol)
Smoking (tobacco, marijuana)
High protein, low carbohydrate diet
Barbecued meat
Childhood

*Decreased clearance*

Enzyme inhibition (cimetidine, erythromycin, ciprofloxacin, allopurinol)
Congestive heart failure
Liver disease
Pneumonia
Viral infection and vaccination
High carbohydrate diet
Old age

needed, although some preparations are designed for once daily administration. For nocturnal asthma a single dose of slow-release theophylline at night is often effective.

Once optimal doses have been determined plasma concentrations usually remain stable, providing no factors which alter clearance change.

Other theophylline salts, such as choline theophyllinate, have no advantages and some derivatives, such as acepiphylline, diprophylline and proxophylline, are less effective. Compound tablets which contain adrenergic agonists and sedatives in addition to theophylline should be avoided.

*Other routes.* Aminophylline may be given as a suppository, but rectal absorption is unreliable and proctitis may occur, so is best avoided. Inhalation of theophylline is irritant and ineffective. Intramuscular injections of theophylline are very painful and should never be given.

### Side-effects

Unwanted effects of theophylline are usually related to plasma concentration and tend to occur when plasma levels exceed 20 mg/l. However, some patients develop side-effects even at low plasma concentrations. To some extent side-effects may be reduced by gradually increasing the dose until therapeutic concentrations are achieved.

The commonest side-effects are headache, nausea and vomiting, abdominal discomfort and restlessness (Box 2.7). There may also be increased acid secretion and diuresis. There has recently been concern that theophylline, even at therapeutic concentrations, may lead to behavioural disturbance and learning difficulties in school children, although it is difficult to design adequate controls for such studies.

At high concentrations convulsions and cardiac arrhythmias may occur. Some of the side-effects (central stimulation, gastric secretion, diuresis and arrhythmias) may be due to adenosine receptor antagonism and may therefore be avoided by drugs such as enprofylline, which has no significant adenosine antagonism at bronchodilator doses.

### Clinical use

In patients with acute asthma intravenous aminophylline is less effective than nebulised $\beta$-agonists, and should therefore be reserved for those patients who fail to respond to $\beta$-agonists.

Theophylline has little or no effect on bronchomotor tone in normal airways, but reverses bronchoconstriction in asthmatic patients, although it is less effective than inhaled $\beta$-agonists and is more likely to have unwanted effects. There is good evidence that theophylline and $\beta$-agonists have additive effects, even if true synergy is not seen, and there is evidence that theophylline may provide an additional bronchodilator effect even when maximally effective doses of $\beta$-agonist have been given. This means that, if adequate bronchodilation is not achieved by a $\beta$-agonist alone, theophylline may be added to the maintenance therapy with benefit. Theophylline may be useful in some patients with nocturnal asthma, since slow-release preparations are able to provide therapeutic concentrations overnight and are more effective than slow-release $\beta$-agonists. Although theophylline is less effective than a $\beta$-agonist and corticosteroids there are a minority of asthmatic patients who appear to derive unexpected benefit, and even patients on oral steroids may show a determination in lung function when theophylline is withdrawn.

---

**Box 2.7  Side-effects of theophylline**

Nausea and vomiting
Gastrointestinal disturbance
Headache
Restlessness
Gastroesophageal reflux
Diuresis
Cardiac arrhythmias
Epileptic seizures
Behavioural disturbance in children (controversial)

Theophylline may also benefit patients with COAD, increasing exercise tolerance, although without any improvement in spirometry tests unless combined with an inhaled $\beta$-agonist. However, theophylline may reduce trapped gas volume, suggesting an effect on peripheral airways, and this may explain why some patients obtain considerable symptomatic improvement.

## ANTI-INFLAMMATORY AGENTS

Inflammation underlies several lung diseases, although the type of inflammatory responses may differ between diseases. Anti-inflammatory drugs suppress the inflammatory response by inhibiting components of the inflammation, such as inflammatory cell infiltration and activation or release, synthesis and effects of inflammatory mediators. Several types of anti-inflammatory drug have been used in the treatment of lung disease.

## Corticosteroids

Corticosteroids are used in the treatment of several lung diseases. They were introduced for the treatment of asthma shortly after their discovery in the 1950s and remain the most effective therapy available for asthma. However, side-effects and fear of adverse effects have limited their use and there has therefore been considerable research into discovering new or related agents which retain the beneficial action on airways without unwanted effects. The introduction of inhaled steroids has been a major advance in the treatment of chronic asthma. Now asthma is viewed as a chronic inflammatory disease, inhaled steroids may even be considered as first-line therapy in all but the mildest of cases. Oral steroids are indicated in the treatment of several other pulmonary diseases, such as sarcoidosis, interstitial lung diseases and pulmonary eosinophilic syndromes.

### Chemistry

The adrenal cortex secretes cortisol (hydrocortisone) and, by modification of its structure, it

was possible to develop derivatives such as prednisolone and dexamethasone with enhanced corticosteroid effects but with reduced mineralocorticoid activity. These derivatives with potent glucocorticoid actions were effective in asthma when given systemically but had no anti-asthmatic activity when given by inhalation. Further substitution in the $17\alpha$ ester position resulted in steroids with high topical activity, such as beclomethasone dipropionate (BDP) and budesonide, which were potent in the skin and were later found to have significant anti-asthma effects when given by

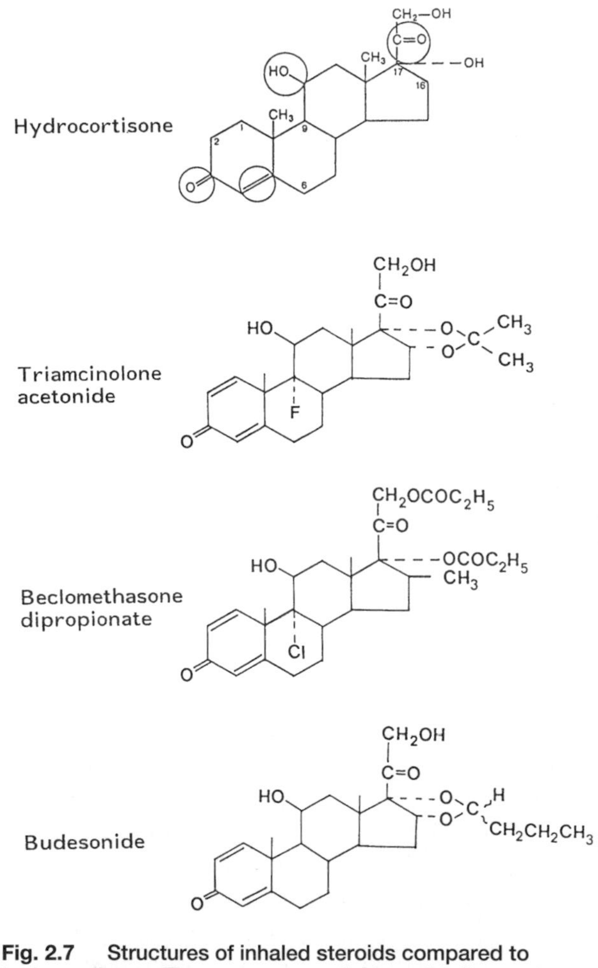

**Fig. 2.7** Structures of inhaled steroids compared to hydrocortisone. The groups essential to anti-inflammatory activity of hydrocortisone are circled.

inhalation (Fig. 2.7). A new inhaled steroid, fluticasone propionate, is currently in clinical trial and appears to have very low bioavailability and may therefore have less systemic effects than BDP when high inhaled doses are required.

The anti-asthma potency of an inhaled steroid is approximately proportional to its anti-inflammatory potency, measured by a skin blanching test. Budesonide has a similar potency to BDP and is 1000 times more potent than prednisolone. More recent studies have shown that, to achieve maximal effects, only short exposure time to a steroid may be necessary, although the effects of the steroid may be slow in onset. This implies that, if topical steroids could be metabolised locally, the full local effect may be obtained but the incidence of systemic side-effects should be reduced, which would allow higher inhaled doses to be administered. Such local metabolism occurs to some extent with both budesonide and BDP, but further improvements may be possible. Budesonide is extensively metabolised in liver and therefore any budesonide swallowed after inhalation will be broken down by first pass metabolism when absorbed from the gut before reaching the systemic circulation. This may be the reason why inhaled budesonide may be less likely to have systemic effects than BDP when high inhaled doses are required.

### Mode of action

*Steroid receptors.* Most steroid effects are mediated by interaction with specific receptors but, at concentrations higher than those used therapeutically, non-specific effects due to insertion into the cell membrane may be seen. Steroids enter target cells and combine with specific receptors within the cytoplasm. These receptors are specific to certain classes of steroids (such as corticosteroids, androgens, oestrogens) but each class is similar in all tissues.

The steroid-receptor complex is transported to the nucleus where it binds to specific sequences on the upstream regulatory element of certain target genes, resulting in increased or decreased transcription of the gene which leads to increased or decreased protein synthesis. This sequence of events may take some time and explains why the onset of steroid effects is usually several hours. However, corticosteroids can have more rapid effects on $Ca^{2+}$ flux and vascular permeability, which may be independent of protein synthesis. Steroid receptors may also interact directly with protein transcription factors in the cytoplasm and thereby influence the synthesis of certain proteins independently of an interaction with DNA in the cell nucleus.

*Lipocortin.* Corticosteroids inhibit the release of arachidonic acid metabolites and PAF from lung and macrophages by the production of a protein called lipocortin, which inhibits phospholipase $A_2$ in the cell membrane. This 37kDa protein has now been cloned and expressed. This provides a unitary hypothesis for the mode of action of steroids through inhibition of phospholipase $A_2$ (and thus the formation of prostaglandins, leukotrienes and PAF). Steroids may also inhibit other phospholipases such as phospholipase C. But it is unlikely that lipocortin can account for many of the antiinflammatory effects of steroids in asthma, and steroids may induce the synthesis of several regulatory proteins through multiple steroid-responsive genes.

*Anti-inflammatory effects.* The mechanism of action of corticosteroids in airway diseases is still poorly understood, but is most likely to be related to their anti-inflammatory properties. There is increasing evidence that asthma and airway hyperresponsiveness are due to an inflammatory process in the airways and there are several components of this inflammatory response which might be inhibited by steroids (Fig. 2.8). Several studies of bronchial biopsies in asthma have demonstrated a reduction in the number and activation of inflammatory cells in the epithelium and submucosa after regular inhaled steroids, together with a healing of the damaged epithelium. Indeed in mild asthmatics the inflammation may be completely resolved after inhaled steroids.

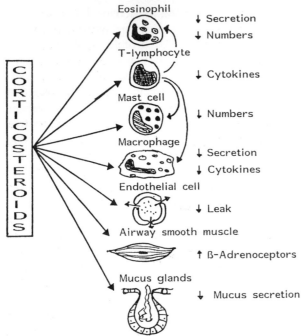

**Fig. 2.8** Effect of steroids on airway inflammatory mechanisms.

Steroids inhibit secretion by human pulmonary macrophages of leukotrienes and prostaglandins, but have no direct action on human lung mast cells. They also cause a fall in circulating eosinophils, inhibit tissue eosinophilia and inhibit degranulation and adherence of eosinophils. In addition, they induce a fall in circulating T-lymphocytes. Steroids potently inhibit the formation of cytokines, such as interleukin (IL)-1, IL-2, IL-3, IL-5 and granulocyte–macrophage colony stimulating factor (GM–CSF) by lymphocytes and macrophages. Indeed this may be the most important action of steroids in suppressing asthmatic inflammation, since cytokines may play a very critical role in the maintenance of the chronic eosinophilic inflammation.

Steroids prevent and reverse the increase in vascular permeability due to inflammatory mediators and may therefore lead to resolution of airway oedema.

*Effect on airway function.* Steroids have no direct effect on airway smooth muscle and improvement in lung function is presumably due to an effect on the chronic airway inflammation and bronchial reactivity. In a single dose inhaled steroids have no effect on the early response to allergen (reflecting their lack of effect on mast cells), but inhibit the late response (which may be due to an effect on macrophages and eosinophils) and also inhibit the increase in airway hyperresponsiveness. Inhaled steroids also reduce airway hyperresponsiveness but this effect may take several weeks or months and presumably reflects the slow healing of the damaged inflamed airway. Steroids have no immediate effect on the early bronchoconstrictor response to allergen or exercise but, if taken over several weeks, there is a reduction even in the acute constrictor responses. This could be due to reduced bronchial responsiveness or due to a reduction in mast cell numbers in airway tissue, which has been demonstrated in the bronchial mucosa after inhaled steroids.

*Effect on β-receptors.* Steroids increase β-adrenergic responsiveness, but whether this is relevant to their effect in asthma is uncertain. Steroids potentiate the effects of β-agonists on bronchial smooth muscle and prevent and reverse β-receptor tachyphylaxis in airways in vitro. In vivo steroids similarly reverse tolerance to β-agonists in dogs and normal man.

Steroids increase the density of β-receptors in rat lung membranes, increase the proportion of receptors in the high affinity binding state in human leukocytes, and reverse and prevent the fall in leukocyte β-receptor density after β-agonists in normal and asthmatic subjects. At a molecular level steroids increase the gene transcription of β-receptors. This action of steroids on β-receptor expression is unlikely to contribute to their anti-asthma effect, but may be clinically important in preventing the development of β-receptor tolerance when high doses of nebulised β-agonists are used.

### Pharmacokinetics

Prednisolone is readily and consistently absorbed after oral administration with little inter-individual variation. Enteric coatings to reduce the incidence of dyspepsia delay absorption but do not affect total amount absorbed. Prednisolone is metabolised in the liver and drugs such as rifampicin, phenobarbitone or phenytoin, which induce hepatic enzymes, lower the plasma half-life of prednisolone. The plasma half-life is 2–3 hours, although its biological half-life is approximately 24 hours, so that it is suitable for daily dosing. There is no evidence that previous exposure to steroids changes their subsequent metabolism. Prednisolone is approximately 92% protein bound, the majority to a specific protein, transcortin, and the remainder to albumin; it is the unbound fraction which is biologically active.

Some patients, usually with severe asthma, apparently fail to respond to corticosteroids. 'Steroid resistant' asthma is not due to impaired absorption or metabolism of steroids and may be associated with a defect in responsiveness of certain cells to steroids.

The pharmacokinetics of inhaled steroids is important in relation to systemic effects. The fraction of steroid which is inhaled into the lungs acts locally on the airway mucosa and may be absorbed from the airway and alveolar surface and therefore reach the systemic circulation. The fraction of inhaled steroid which is deposited in the oropharynx is swallowed and absorbed from the gut. The absorbed fraction may be metabolised in the liver before reaching the systemic circulation. Budesonide has a greater first pass metabolism than BDP and is therefore less likely to produce systemic effects at high inhaled doses. The use of a large volume spacer chamber reduces oropharyngeal deposition and therefore reduces systemic absorption of steroids. Similarly rinsing the mouth and discarding the rinse has a similar effect and this procedure should be used with high dose dry powder steroid inhalers, since spacer chambers cannot be used with these devices.

### Routes of administration

*Oral.* Prednisolone or prednisone are the most commonly used steroids. Prednisone is converted to prednisolone in the liver.

Clinical improvement with oral steroids may take several days and the maximal beneficial effect is usually achieved with 30–40 mg prednisone daily, although a few patients may need 60 mg daily to achieve control of symptoms. The usual maintenance dose is in the order of 10–15 mg/day.

Oral steroids should be given in a single dose in the morning, since this coincides with the normal diurnal increase in plasma cortisol and there is therefore less adrenal suppression than if given in divided doses or at night. Furthermore, the amount of steroid bound to transcortin is less during the day, resulting in higher free concentrations, and this might contribute to the greater functional effect. Although steroids are traditionally given as a single morning dose there is some evidence that they are more effective in the control of asthma if given in the afternoon, and it may be worth switching to this dosing regime if asthma proves difficult to control.

Alternate day treatment has advantages, since there is less adrenal suppression and other side-effects with similar control of asthma, although some patients' control is not optimal on this regime.

*Intravenous.* Parenteral steroids are indicated in acute severe exacerbations of asthma. Hydrocortisone is the steroid of choice as it has the most rapid onset (5–6 hours after administration), being more rapid than prednisolone (8 hours). The dose required is still uncertain, but it is common to give hydrocortisone 4 mg/kg initially followed by a maintenance dose of 3 mg/kg/6 hours. These doses are based on the argument that it is necessary to maintain 'stress' levels of plasma cortisol.

*Inhaled.* Inhaled topical steroids have been a great advance in the management of chronic asthma as it may be possible to control symptoms without adrenal suppression or side-effects, and allows a reduction in the dose of oral maintenance steroids. The high topical activity of inhaled steroids means that only small doses are required and any swallowed drug is immediately metabolised by the liver. Only when much larger doses are inhaled is sufficient steroid absorbed to cause adrenal suppression.

Many patients get a maximal response at a dose of 400–500 μg per day, but some patients may benefit from higher doses (up to 2000 μg/day) and high dose inhalers have therefore been introduced. Traditionally steroid inhalers have been used 4 times daily, but twice daily administration is usually as effective and compliance is likely to be better.

Several inhaled preparations are available, including beclomethasone dipropionate (BDP), budesonide, triamcinolone and flunisolide (Table 2.2). Fluticasone propionate, which has a low oral bioavailability, has recently become available in some countries.

### Side-effects

*Adrenal suppression.* Steroids inhibit ACTH and cortisol secretion by a negative feedback effect on the pituitary gland. This suppression is dependent on dose, and usually only occurs when a dose of prednisolone greater than 7.5–10 mg daily is used. Significant suppression after short courses of steroid therapy is not usually a problem, but prolonged suppression may occur after several months or years. Steroid doses after prolonged oral therapy must therefore be reduced slowly. Symptoms of 'steroid withdrawal syndrome' include lassitude, musculoskeletal pains and occasionally fever.

*Systemic side-effects.* Side-effects of long-term corticosteroid therapy are well described and include fluid retention, increased appetite, weight gain, osteroporosis, capillary fragility, hypertension, peptic ulceration, diabetes, cataracts and psychosis. Their frequency tends to increase with age. Very occasionally adverse reactions (such as anaphylaxis) to intravenous hydrocortisone have been described, particularly in aspirin-sensitive asthmatics.

The incidence of systemic side-effects after inhaled steroids is an important consideration (Box 2.8). Initial studies suggested that adrenal suppression only occurred when inhaled doses of over 1500–2000 μg daily were used. More sensitive measurements of systemic effects include indices of bone metabolism, such as serum osteocalcin and urinary hydroxyproline excretion which may be increased with inhaled doses as low as 400 μg in some patients. The clinical relevance of these measurements is not yet clear however. Nevertheless it is important

| Table 2.2 | Inhaled steroids | |
|---|---|---|
| **Drug** | **Trade Name** | **Dose** (μg/puff) |
| Beclomethasone dipropionate | Becotide | MDI: 50, 100 Rotacaps: 100, 200, 400 |
| | Becloforte | MDI: 250 |
| | Becodisks | 100, 200, 400 |
| Budesonide | Pulmicort | MDI: 50, 200 Turbohaler: 200, 400 |
| Betamethasone maleate | Bextasol | MDI: 100 |
| Triamcinolone acetonide | Not available in the UK | |
| Flunisolide | Not available in the UK | |
| Fluticasone propionate | Flixotide | Diskhaler: 50, 100, 200 |

to reduce the likelihood of systemic effects by using the lowest dose of inhaled steroid needed to control the asthma, by the use of a large volume spacer to reduce oropharyngeal deposition (and therefore the fraction absorbed from the gastrointestinal tract), and by using budesonide in preference to BDP when high doses of inhaled steroids are needed.

There has been concern about the use of inhaled steroids in children because of growth suppression. Most studies have been reassuring in that doses of 400 μg or less have not been associated with impaired growth, and there may even be a growth spurt as asthma is better controlled.

*Local side-effects.* Side-effects of inhaled steroids are few. The most common problem is hoarseness and weakness of the voice (dysphonia) which is due to laryngeal deposition. It may occur in up to 40% of patients and is noticed particularly by patients who need to use their voices during their work (lecturers, teachers and singers). It may be due to atrophy of the vocal cords. Throat irritation and coughing after inhalation are common with MDIs and appear to be due to the additives, since these problems are not usually seen if the patient switches to the dry powder inhalers. Oropharyngeal candidiasis may occur in 5% of patients. The incidence of local side-effects may be related to the local concentrations of steroid deposited and may be reduced by the use of large volume spacers, which markedly reduce oropharyngeal deposition. Local side-effects are also less likely when inhaled steroids are used twice daily rather than four times daily.

There is no evidence for atrophy of the lining of the airway, or of an increase in lung infections (including tuberculosis) after inhaled steroids.

## Clinical use

*Acute asthma.* Hydrocortisone is given intravenously in acute asthma. While the value of corticosteroids in acute severe asthma has been questioned, others have found that they speed the resolution of attacks. There is no apparent

---

**Box 2.8 Side-effects of inhaled steroids**

*Local side-effects*
Hoarseness (dysphonia)
Oropharyngeal candidiasis
Throat irritation and cough (due to additives)

*Systemic side-effects*
Adrenal suppression
Easy bruising
Skin thinning
Increased bone metabolism, osteoporosis
Cataracts
Stunted growth in children
Behavioural disturbances?

---

advantage in giving very high doses of intravenous steroids (such as methylprednisolone 1 g). Intravenous steroids are indicated in acute asthma if lung function is less than 30% predicted and where there is no significant improvement with nebulised β-agonist. Intravenous therapy is usually given until a satisfactory response is obtained and then oral prednisolone may be substituted. Oral prednisolone (40–60 mg) has a similar effect to intravenous hydrocortisone and is easier to administer. Inhaled steroids have no proven effect in acute asthma, but trials with nebulised steroids are underway.

### Chronic asthma

Inhaled steroids are now recommended as first-line therapy for all but the mildest of asthmatic patients. Inhaled steroids should be started in any patient who needs to use a β-agonist inhaler for symptom control once a day or more frequently. Oral steroids are reserved for patients who cannot be controlled on other therapy, the dose being titrated to the lowest which provides acceptable control of symptoms. For any patient taking regular oral steroids objective evidence of steroid responsiveness should be obtained before maintenance therapy is instituted.

Short courses of oral steroids (such as 30 mg prednisolone daily for 1–2 weeks) are indicated for exacerbations of asthma, and the dose may be tailed off over 1 week once the exacerbation is resolved (although the tail-off period is not strictly necessary patients find it reassuring).

For most patients inhaled steroids should be used twice daily, which improves compliance, once control of asthma has been achieved (which may require 4-times daily dosing initially). If a dose of more than 800 $\mu$g daily is used a spacer device should be used as this reduces the risk of oropharyngeal side-effects. Inhaled steroids may be used in children in the same way as adults and at doses of 400 $\mu$g daily or less there is no evidence of growth suppression.

*Chronic bronchitis.* Chronic bronchitis patients occasionally respond to steroids and these patients are likely to be undiagnosed asthmatics. Steroids have no objective benefit of airway function in patients with true chronic bronchitis, although they may often produce subjective benefit because of their euphoric effect. It is not yet certain whether the use of inhaled steroids delays the progressive fall in lung function seen in patients with COAD and large-scale clinical trials to answer this important question are now underway.

## Sodium cromoglycate

Sodium cromoglycate (SCG) is a derivative of khellin, an Egyptian herbal remedy which was found to protect against allergen challenge without bronchodilator effect. It is classified as a chromone.

### Mode of action

*Mast cell stabilisation.* Initial investigations indicated that SCG inhibited the release of mediators by allergen in passively sensitised human and animal lung, and inhibited passive cutaneous anaphylaxis in rat, although it was without effect in guinea pig. This activity was attributed to stabilisation of the mast cell membrane and thus SCG was classified as a mast cell stabiliser. However, SCG has a rather low potency in stabilising human lung mast cells, and other drugs which are more potent in this respect have little or no effect in clinical asthma. This has raised doubts about mast cell stabilisation as the mode of action of SCG.

*Interaction with sensory nerves.* SCG potently inhibits bronchoconstriction induced by sulphur dioxide and bradykinin, which are believed to act through activation of sensory nerves in the airway. In dogs, SCG suppresses firing of unmyelinated C-fibre nerve endings, reinforcing the view that it might be acting to suppress sensory nerve activation and thus neurogenic inflammation in airways.

*Effect on other inflammatory cells.* SCG has variable inhibitory actions on other inflammatory cells which may participate in allergic inflammation, including macrophages and eosinophils. In vivo SCG is capable of blocking the early response to allergen (which may be mediated by mast cells) but also the late response and airway hyperresponsiveness, which are more likely to be mediated by macrophage and eosinophil interactions.

### Administration

SCG is not lipid soluble and is not significantly absorbed after oral administration. It must be delivered by inhalation, either as a dry powder or as a metered dose inhaler. There is little information about dose–response relationships and the doses used in clinical practice are somewhat arbitrary.

### Side-effects

SCG is one of the safest drugs available and side-effects are extremely rare. The dry powder inhaler may cause throat irritation, coughing and, occasionally, wheezing but this is usually prevented by prior administration of a $\beta$-agonist inhaler.

Very rarely a transient rash and urticaria are seen and a few cases of pulmonary eosinophilia have been reported, all of which are due to hypersensitivity.

### Clinical use

SCG is a prophylactic treatment and needs to be given regularly. SCG protects against various indirect bronchoconstrictor stimuli, such as exercise and fog. It is only effective in mild asthma, but does not appear to be effective in all patients and there seems no sure way of predicting which patients are likely to respond. SCG is often the anti-inflammatory drug of first choice in children because it has almost no side-effects. In adults, steroids by inhalation are preferred as they are effective in all patients, although adults with mild asthma do respond to SCG. SCG has to be given 4 times daily to provide good protection, which makes it less useful than inhaled steroids which may be given twice daily. It may also be taken prior to exercise in children with exercise-induced asthma that is not blocked by an inhaled $\beta$-agonist.

## Other anti-allergic drugs

SCG is classified as an anti-allergic drug in the belief that it has a specific effect on allergic inflammation. This was originally viewed as an effect on mast cells, but now it is clear that other inflammatory cells are also involved. Several other drugs may also be included in this category.

### Nedocromil sodium

Nedocromil sodium (NS) is a new prophylactic drug which has a similar profile of activity to SCG. It is more potent in various challenge tests and may have a longer duration of action. In clinical practice NS has a very similar efficacy to SCG and is therefore indicated in patients with mild asthma. There is some evidence that it may have steroid sparing effects and therefore may be considered as a means of reducing the dose of inhaled steroid needed to control asthma when local side-effects are a problem.

Side effects are not usually a problem although some patients have noticed a sensation of flushing after using the inhaler. Many patients find the bitter taste unpleasant, but a menthol flavoured version is now available which seems to overcome this problem.

### Ketotifen

Ketotifen is described as a prophylactic anti-asthma compound. Its predominant effect is $H_1$-receptor antagonism and it is this antihistaminic effect which accounts for its sedative effect. Ketotifen has little effect in clinical asthma, either in acute challenge, on airway hyperresponsiveness or on clinical symptoms. A long-term placebo control trial of oral ketotifen in children with mild asthma showed no clinical benefit.

### Antihistamines

$H_1$-receptor antagonists block the bronchoconstrictor effect of histamine and, if histamine released from airway mast cells contributes to the features of asthma, then antihistamines should be beneficial. Antihistamines were previously limited in the dose which could be given because of side-effects such as drowsiness. *Non-sedating* antihistamines, such as terfenadine, loratidine and astemizole, have been introduced. These antihistamines are useful in treating the symptoms of allergic rhinitis and reduce the early bronchoconstrictor response to allergen and exercise (in which mast cell degranulation is involved), but are not useful in the treatment of chronic asthma, presumably because other mediators are more important.

### Mast cell stabilisers

Almost 40 drugs have now been developed as 'mast cell stabilisers'. In vitro these drugs inhibit mast cell mediator release triggered by allergen but all of these drugs have been disappointing in the treatment of clinical asthma, and none have become available for clinical use. Presumably this reflects the fact that mast cells do not play a prominent role in the inflammatory response of chronic asthma.

### Cyclo-oxygenase inhibitors

Aspirin and other non-steroidal anti-inflammatory agents, by inhibiting the formation of prostaglandins and thromboxane, may theoretically be useful in the treatment of asthma. In practice they have not been found to produce beneficial effects and in a small number of asthmatics (aspirin-sensitive asthmatics) may precipitate bronchoconstriction.

### Immunotherapy

There is little sound evidence that desensitising injections to common allergens are very effective in controlling chronic asthma, although they do have some effectiveness in rhinitis. Because there is a risk of anaphylactic and local reactions, and because the course of treatment is time consuming, this form of therapy is not recommended. In the future more specific vaccines may be developed which are more effective.

## Immunosuppressive therapy

Immunosuppressive therapy (in addition to steroids) has been considered in asthma when other treatments have been unsuccessful or to reduce the dose of oral steroids required.

### Methotrexate

Low dose methotrexate (15 mg weekly) has been shown to have a steroid-sparing effect in asthma and may be indicated when oral steroids are contraindicated because of unacceptable side-effects (e.g. in postmenopausal women when osteoporosis is a problem). However side-effects are relatively common and include nausea (reduced if methotrexate is given as a weekly *injection*), blood dyscrasias and hepatic damage. Careful monitoring of such patients (monthly blood counts and liver enzymes) is essential. Closer analysis of the studies which have reported a beneficial effect suggest that while the mean sparing amounts to 5–7 mg prednisolone, there are some patients in whom a much greater sparing effect is observed. It may also be necessary to administer methotrexate over 6 months before beneficial effects are apparent.

### Gold

Gold has long been used in the treatment of chronic arthritis. There is anecdotal evidence that it may also be useful in asthma, and it has been used in Japan for many years. An open study showed some efficacy of an oral gold preparation (auranofin) in chronic asthma, and this has been confirmed in a recent double-blind study indicating that auranofin has a small steroid-sparing effect (equivalent to about 5 mg prednisolone).

### Cyclosporin A

Cyclosporin A is active against CD4+ lymphocytes and might therefore be useful in asthma, in which these cells are implicated. Trials of cyclosporin A in patients with steroid-dependent asthma indicate that it can improve control of symptoms in patients with severe asthma on oral steroids and may allow a reduction of steroids. Like methotrexate cyclosporin appears to benefit some patients more than others. Its use is likely to be limited by side-effects, such as nephrotoxicity and hypertension.

## CLINICAL APPLICATION

## Asthma

Despite a marked increase in treatments prescribed for asthma the morbidity and even mortality are increasing in industrialised countries, against the trend for other common treatable conditions. This may be related to inappropriate use of available medication or to a lack of appropriate therapies.

### Management guidelines

The aim of asthma management is to allow patients to lead as normal a life as possible, including participation in sport, to reduce the frequency and severity of exacerbations and to achieve this control with minimal side-effects.

General measures include *allergen avoidance*, where this is practical. This is particularly important in occupational asthma. Improvements in drug therapy for asthma now mean that it is possible to obtain good control of asthma in most patients if the treatments are used correctly. There are rather few categories of drug available for asthma therapy (Fig. 2.9). In several countries guidelines for the treatment of asthma have now been introduced. These are based on the understanding that asthma is an inflammatory disease and stress the early introduction of anti-inflammatory treatments. The guidelines outline a stepwise approach to therapy with increasing therapies depending on the response to treatment (Fig. 2.10).

*Step 1: inhaled $\beta_2$-agonist as required.* For patients with only occasional symptoms an inhaled $\beta_2$ agonist should be used when necessary, and never on a regular basis.

*Step 2: low-dose anti-inflammatory treatment.* For patients with more frequent symptoms (e.g. daily) some form of prophylactic treatment should be considered. Either low-dose inhaled steroids or SCG/NS should be introduced in addition to an inhaled $\beta_2$-agonist, which should only be taken on demand for symptom control. SCG is often tried before inhaled steroids in children, but if it is ineffective after 1 month then low-dose inhaled steroids should be introduced.

*Step 3: high-dose inhaled steroids.* If satisfactory control is not achieved then the dose of inhaled steroid should be increased. It is often useful to start with a moderate dose of inhaled steroids (such as 800 $\mu$g daily) until the asthma is controlled and then to reduce the dose gradually until the minimum necessary dose is found. This strategy has the advantage of achieving more rapid control of the disease. Doses of up to 1.5–2 mg daily may be given before systemic effects of adrenocortical suppression are seen. However some patients appear to be more susceptible to the systemic effects of inhaled steroids and such side-effects (thinning of the skin, weight increase, ecchymoses) should be sought.

Inhaled steroids should be given 4 times daily until control is achieved, but may then be given twice daily as this gives better compliance. For doses of over 800 $\mu$g daily a large volume spacer device should be used to reduce the risk of oropharyngeal side-effects.

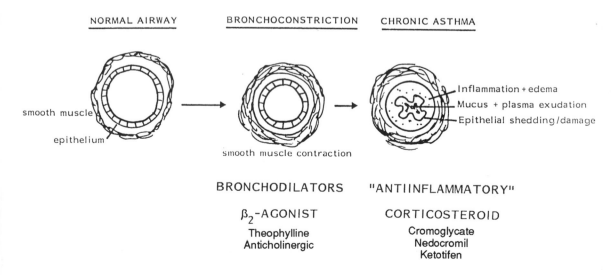

**Fig. 2.9** Drugs currently used for asthma therapy.

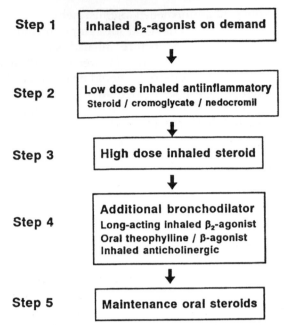

**Step 1** — Inhaled β₂-agonist on demand

**Step 2** — Low dose inhaled antiinflammatory
Steroid / cromoglycate / nedocromil

**Step 3** — High dose inhaled steroid

**Step 4** — Additional bronchodilator
Long-acting inhaled β₂-agonist
Oral theophylline / β-agonist
Inhaled anticholinergic

**Step 5** — Maintenance oral steroids

**Fig. 2.10** Example of an action plan to treat exacerbation of asthma.

*Step 4: additional bronchodilators.* Theophylline, given as a slow-release preparation, may be added as a third-line treatment and the dose must be carefully monitored to give therapeutic plasma concentrations as indicated previously. If theophylline is considered as a treatment the patient should be under the care of a specialist.

Long-acting inhaled β-agonists, such as salmeterol, may also be added when asthma is not controlled by inhaled steroids up to doses of 1000 μg daily. Long-acting inhaled β-agonists should always be used as a fixed twice daily dosage and short-acting inhaled β-agonists, such as salbutamol, used as rescue therapy.

Anticholinergic drugs usually have little beneficial effect in chronic asthma, but they are worth trying, preferably with peak flow monitoring to determine any objective benefit. They seem to be more useful in elderly patients in whom there may be an element of COAD.

*Step 5: maintenance oral steroids.* When asthma is more difficult to control it may be necessary to introduce oral steroids. Prednisone or prednisolone are the treatments of choice and

the lowest dose which controls the symptoms should be used in order to avoid long-term complications. Oral steroids should be given as a single dose in the morning as this reduces the side-effects. Alternate day dosing, while reducing side-effects, gives less satisfactory control. In some patients who have particular problems with oral steroids (e.g. osteoporosis in postmenopausal women) low-dose oral methotrexate (15 mg/week) and low-dose cyclosporin A may be useful in sparing the oral steroid dose.

The control of asthma should be monitored by recording of peak flow. The inflammation of asthma is variable, which means that the doses of anti-asthma treatments can be varied from time to time. The frequency of use of β₂-agonists by inhalation gives a rough guide to adequacy of control and, if this increases, then the amount of prophylactic treatment given should be increased until control is achieved.

### Exacerbations

Exacerbations of asthma should be dealt with by a short course of oral steroids (e.g. prednisolone 30–40 mg daily for 2 weeks). Less severe exacerbations may be treated by doubling the dose of inhaled steroids. Patients with more severe chronic asthma should be given a *crisis management plan* (Fig. 2.11), indicating when they should have a course of oral steroids, based on the measurement of peak flow at home. Such self-administered treatment has been shown to reduce hospital admissions and is acceptable to patients.

### Severe acute asthma

Severe exacerbations of asthma usually respond to high-dose nebulised β₂-agonists (Box 2.9). Less severe episodes may be managed at home using a nebuliser or a large volume spacer device.

More severe episodes require hospital admission. Nebulised β₂-agonist (e.g. salbutamol 5 mg in 2 ml saline nebulised over 10 min) is the initial treatment of choice and is more convenient and as effective as intravenous β₂-agonist. The

# ACTION PLAN FOR EXACERBATIONS

- **Measure PEF every morning (more frequently if unstable)**

---

- **If PEF falls to <70% normal: double inhaled steroids**

- **If PEF falls to <50% normal: course of oral steroids**

- **If PEF falls to <30% normal: medical attention needed**

**Fig. 2.11** Stepwise approach to chronic asthma therapy.

nebuliser should be driven by oxygen to avoid the fall in $Po_2$ which may occur from the associated pulmonary vasodilation. If there is no response the nebulisation should be repeated within 20 min. Nebulisation should be repeated 3–4 hourly. If there is a poor response to the initial nebulisation with $\beta$-agonist, nebulised ipratropium bromide (0.5–1 mg) should be added to the second nebulisation of $\beta$-agonist, as there is evidence for an additional bronchodilatation without increased side-effects. Ipratropium bromide should not be used alone as there is a risk of paradoxical bronchoconstriction (although this is less now that additives have been removed from the nebulised preparation) and it has a relatively slow onset of action.

Intravenous aminophylline is more difficult to use and may be associated with unwanted effects. A theophylline blood level should be measured before starting and, if the patient was taking a theophylline preparation, the dose of aminophylline should be reduced accordingly. Aminophylline should only be used if the patient fails to respond satisfactorily to nebulised $\beta$-agonist and anticholinergic (which is rare). Steroids should be given to all patients with acute severe asthma. Intravenous hydrocortisone (200 mg 6 hourly) is usually given, but prednisolone 40–60 mg orally is just as effective unless the patient is very ill (and therefore has impaired gastric absorption).

Careful monitoring is necessary in all patients who have been admitted with acute severe asthma. Patients should be changed from nebulised bronchodilators to regular inhalers well before discharge from hospital and should be given a crisis management plan which clearly indicates when oral steroids should be introduced, based on daily measurement of peak flow.

### Exercise-induced asthma

Exercise-induced asthma is a sign of poor control and usually responds to an increase in inhaled steroids. Inhalation of a $\beta_2$-agonist or inhaled SCG 10 minutes prior to exercise usually prevents exercise-induced wheeze. Anticholinergics, theophylline and oral $\beta$-agonists are less satisfactory. Long-acting inhaled $\beta_2$-agonists may be the most suitable prophylactic treatment in view of the long duration of protection against bronchoconstriction provided.

### Nocturnal asthma

Nocturnal wheezing reflects poor control of asthma and usually responds to improved control with inhaled steroids. If nocturnal symptoms persist, even with high-dose inhaled steroids, a slow-release theophylline preparation at night may be helpful. Slow-release oral

$\beta$-agonists may also be useful in some patients. Long-acting inhaled $\beta_2$-agonists may be the treatment of choice when nocturnal asthma persists in spite of a dose of inhaled steroids of 1000 $\mu$g daily.

## Difficult asthma

Occasionally, asthma may remain difficult to control, despite seemingly adequate treatment. This is often related to poor compliance, which should be carefully checked (Box 2.10). Sometimes the diagnosis is incorrect (cardiac failure, very rarely carcinoid syndrome). Some patients have vocal cord dysfunction which presents as asthma but is a conversion (hysterical) syndrome.

Some patients have 'brittle' asthma, which is unpredictable. Some of these patients respond to subcutaneous infusions of a $\beta_2$-agonist.

Other patients are 'steroid-resistant', and do

---

**Box 2.10   Difficult asthma**

Poor compliance with therapy
Incorrect diagnosis
Unidentified trigger factors (gastroesophageal reflux,  occupational sensitisers, unidentified allergen exposure)
Drugs ($\beta$-blockers, aspirin)
Vocal cord dysfunction
'Brittle' asthma
Steroid-resistant asthma
Premenstrual asthma

---

not respond to even high doses of oral steroids, although they may still have a bronchodilator response. In some of these patients there may be a problem with absorption of the steroids and there are reports of such patients who have responded to triamcinolone injections. Patients with true steroid resistance may have some cellular defect, the nature of which is not clear.  These patients are difficult to manage but methotrexate and cyclosporin A may be tried.

A variant of steroid-resistant asthma is severe *premenstrual* asthma which may respond to high-dose parenteral progesterone.

## Asthma in infants

Children under 2 years may be difficult to manage as inhaled drugs are difficult to administer. Infants do not respond well to $\beta$-agonists and anticholinergics are the most useful bronchodilators at this age. They may be delivered by MDI into a spacer device fitted with a face mask. For severe exacerbations a course of oral steroids and nebulised ipratropium bromide may be given. Recent evidence suggests that nebulised budesonide may also be useful; a relatively high dose must be given as nebulisation is relatively inefficient due to the small tidal breaths.

## Asthma in pregnancy

Asthma often improves during pregnancy, although a few patients may deteriorate. The principles of treatment are the same as for non-

---

**Box 2.9   Management of acute severe asthma**

*Immediate treatment*

Oxygen: highest concentration available
Nebulised $\beta_2$-agonist: salbutamol (5 mg), terbutaline (10 mg)
High-dose systemic steroids: prednisolone 30–60 mg orally
      (hydrocortisone 200 mg i.v. if oral drugs contraindicated)

*If life-threatening features present*

Add ipratropium bromide (0.5 mg) to nebulised $\beta$-agonist
Give i.v. aminophylline (250 mg over 20 min)

*Subsequent management*

Continue oxygen
Continue systemic steroids
If improving continue nebulised $\beta_2$-agonist every 4h.
If *not* improving: give nebulised $\beta_2$-agonist more frequently (up to every 15 min)
      add ipratropium bromide to nebuliser
      consider aminophylline infusion (0.5-0.9 mg/kg/h)
      consider salbutamol (12.5 $\mu$g/min) infusion

*Unhelpful treatments*

All sedation is contraindicated
Only give antibiotics if bacterial infection present
Percussive physiotherapy unnecessary

pregnant asthmatics. Inhaled treatments should be used and inhaled $\beta$-agonists, corticosteroids and SCG are all safe; oral medication should be avoided whenever possible. Oral steroids have been associated with cleft palate when given in the first trimester but the evidence is not very convincing and most anti-asthma medications have a safe record. The major concern should be to control the asthma well, since fetal hypoxia is a much greater risk than any problems with the effect of asthma therapy on fetal development.

# COAD

## General measures

The aims of management and treatment are to treat infective exacerbations promptly, to alleviate symptoms and to prevent complications. For patients with mild symptoms smoking should be stopped, since this will reduce the progressive decline in lung function. Influenza vaccination is recommended in the autumn.

## Acute exacerbations

Acute exacerbations associated with purulent sputum are usually due to *Haemophilus influenzae* or *Streptococcus pneumoniae* and should be treated promptly with a broad spectrum antibiotic, such as amoxycillin or cotrimoxazole. Sputum culture is not helpful in deciding which antibiotic to use and more expensive antibiotics, such as cephalosporins, are rarely indicated.

## Bronchodilator treatment

The degree of bronchodilatation seen in patients with COAD is generally considerably less than in patients with asthma. Inhaled $\beta_2$-agonists and inhaled anticholinergics are the bronchodilators of choice. The only reversible element in patients with COAD is cholinergic tone and therefore both anticholinergics (which are specific) and $\beta$-agonists (which also reverse cholinergic tone) are equally effective. In some patients anticholinergics appear to be more

effective, for reasons which are not clear. Because airflow obstruction is often very marked in COAD patients (with $FEV_1$ values of less than 1 l), only a very small proportion (less than 1% of dose) enters the lung. For this reason home nebulisers are a useful way of delivering larger doses of these agents in some patients. Theophylline is a poor bronchodilator, but has been found useful in patients with COAD for increasing the walking distance, and this may be due to deflation of the hyperinflated lungs, possibly due to a selective action on peripheral airways. Furthermore, theophylline might have an effect on respiratory muscles which increases ventilatory efficiency, although whether this occurs in therapeutic doses is now questioned. It should be noted that, in patients who continue to smoke, the dose of theophylline may need to be higher in order to achieve therapeutic plasma concentrations.

## Oxygen

Controlled oxygen is needed to correct hypoxaemia during acute exacerbations. In hypercapnic patients only low concentrations should be used initially because of the fear of depressing respiratory drive. Domiciliary oxygen, best supplied by an oxygen concentrator, is also indicated in patients with very severe COAD where hypoxaemia limits daily activity. Some measure of objective improvement should be demonstrated, however, before this treatment is instituted.

## Mucolytics and antitussives

Patients with chronic bronchitis commonly have a chronic productive cough. The production of sputum usually decreases when the patient stops smoking. There is no evidence that currently available mucolytic drugs are of any benefit in clearing mucus. Antitussives are not indicated, since coughing is useful in clearing the respiratory tract. Furthermore, opiates may impair ventilatory drive and should be avoided.

### Anti-inflammatory drugs

There is no convincing evidence that corticosteroids, or any other anti-inflammatory treatment, are useful in the chronic management of COAD. Indeed, if a patient shows an improvement with steroids it is safe to assume he is asthmatic and should be treated accordingly. A formal *trial of steroids* (oral prednisolone 30–40 mg daily for 2 weeks) is indicated if there is doubt about the diagnosis, with measurement of peak expiratory flow at home to demonstrate an objective improvement. Several trials to determine whether long-term use of inhaled steroids prevents the accelerated decline in lung function are now underway.

### Drugs for breathlessness

Bronchodilators should reduce breathlessness and chronic oxygen may have some effect, but in a few patients breathlessness may be extreme. Drugs which have been shown to reduce breathlessness may also depress ventilation in parallel. Some patients show a beneficial response to dihydrocodeine and diazepam but these drugs must be used with caution.

### Cor pulmonale

Pulmonary hypertension may develop as a result of chronic hypoxaemia and the progressive destruction of the pulmonary vascular bed in emphysema. This may lead to right-heart failure, fluid retention and peripheral oedema.

Pulmonary hypertension may be reduced by long-term domiciliary oxygen, although it may be necessary to take this for over 15 hours daily). Pulmonary hypertension may also be reduced by various vasodilators (see Ch. 3 for further details).

Peripheral oedema responds to diuretics. Care should be taken with potassium losing diuretics, since this may exacerbate any hypokalaemia induced by large doses of nebulised $\beta$-agonist. Potassium sparing diuretics, or combinations, are preferable. Digoxin is not indicated as oedema is due to fluid retention rather than heart failure and patients with hypoxaemia may be more prone to develop digoxin-induced arrhythmias.

### $\alpha_1$-protease inhibitor therapy

The gene for $\alpha_1$-protease inhibitor ($\alpha_1$-PI) has now been cloned and human recombinant $\alpha_1$-PI has been synthesised. This is likely to be preferable to the same protein extracted from pooled human serum. Trials are now underway in patients with homozygous $\alpha_1$-PI deficiency and is unlikely to be applicable to most patients with emphysema due to smoking.

## DRUGS CONTRAINDICATED IN AIRWAY DISEASE

Several drugs may cause a deterioration in asthma or airway disease.

## Sedatives

Any sedative (opiate, benzodiazepine) may reduce ventilatory drive and should therefore be avoided in patients with COAD and with severe asthma.

## $\beta$-blockers

All $\beta$-blockers should be avoided in patients with asthma. The mechanisms by which $\beta$-blockers impair airway function is not yet certain, but it appears to be mediated by antagonism of $\beta_2$-receptors, although even selective $\beta_1$-blockers are potentially dangerous. Even low doses of $\beta$-blockers, such as timolol eye drops, can cause severe worsening of asthma, and fatalities continue to be reported. The effect is likely to be mediated via airway cholinergic nerves and may be very severe. Patients with COAD are less likely to be affected by $\beta$-blockers, but if they are unrecognised asthmatics these drugs are best avoided. Alternative treatments for hypertension and ischaemic heart disease include calcium channel blockers and $\alpha$-adrenoceptor antagonists which are safe.

Propafenone is a new anti-arrhythmic agent which is structurally similar to propranolol and has been reported to increase bronchoconstriction in asthmatic patients.

## Aspirin

A small proportion of asthmatics (3–5%) develop a worsening of asthma with aspirin. These patients usually have late-onset asthma and also have rhinitis and nasal polyps. Other non-steroidal anti-inflammatory drugs may have similar effects in these patients, suggesting that cyclo-oxygenase inhibition underlies the phenomenon. It is possible that blocking the formation of bronchodilator prostaglandins (such as $PGE_2$) is the critical factor in such patients. Recent evidence suggests that cyclo-oxygenase inhibition may result in increased formation of leukotrienes in such patients, leading to bronchoconstriction.

## ACE inhibitors

Angiotensin converting enzyme (ACE) inhibitors, such as captopril and enalapril, may cause an irritating non-productive cough in approximately 10% of patients treated with ACE inhibitors. This may occur in any patient and is no more frequent in patients with asthma, nor is there any convining evdence that asthma gets worse, although a few cases of asthma exacerbation have been reported. The mechanism of the cough is not certain, but may be due to reduced degradation of certain peptides such as bradykinin. Non-steroidal anti-inflammatory drugs appear to be useful in inhibiting the cough, suggesting that prostaglandins released by endogenous bradykinin are responsible.

## NEW DRUGS

There are now many new drugs under development for the treatment of asthma. Some have now reached the stage of clinical trials, whereas others are in an experimental phase. Some of the new drugs represent an improvement on existing drugs, whereas others are novel compounds (Box 2.11).

## Long-acting inhaled $\beta_2$-agonists

Inhaled $\beta_2$-agonists with a much longer duration of bronchodilator action have recently been introduced in some countries. Both salmeterol and formoterol bronchodilate for over 12 hours and give long-lasting protection against bronchial challenge. Preliminary studies show that they are safe in clinical practice and that tolerance does not develop. They should provide excellent control of asthma symptoms, particularly nocturnal asthma, and are recommended twice daily as maintenance treatment. It is very important to give inhaled steroids in any patient who uses these long-acting $\beta_2$-agonists, as they may not have significant anti-inflammatory effects, and may therefore mask airway inflammation. It is sensible to add long-acting inhaled $\beta_2$-agonists in patients taking 800 $\mu$g inhaled steroid daily in whom symptoms (particularly nocturnal symptoms) persist. These drugs will also be useful as maintenance bronchodilatation in COAD. One relative disadvantage is their high cost.

## Potassium channel activators

Potassium ($K^+$) channels are involved in recovery of excitable cells after depolarisation and therefore are important in stabilisation of cells. $K^+$ channel activators such as cromakalim or lemakalim (the L-isomer of cromakalim) open $K^+$ channels in smooth muscle and therefore relax airway smooth muscle. Preliminary clinical studies suggest that cromakalim, given in a single oral dose at night, has a small protective effect against nocturnal asthma. The cardiovascular side-effects of these drugs (hypotension) may limit the oral dose, however. Perhaps inhaled $K^+$ channel openers may be more useful in the future.

## Selective phosphodiesterase inhibitors

Phosphodiesterase (PDE) breaks down cyclic AMP and, if inhibited, causes cyclic AMP to increase, leading to bronchodilatation. It is now recognised that there are several isoenzymes of PDE which may be selectively inhibited. In human airway smooth muscle type III and type IV isoenzymes are important in relaxation and thus selective inhibitors may be useful bronchodilators. Since type IV isoenzyme is also important in inhibition of inflammatory cells, such drugs may have additional anti-inflammatory effects.

## Mediator antagonists/inhibitors

Several lipid mediators have been implicated in asthma and recently potent antagonists have been developed to some of these mediators.

Leukotrienes have long been implicated in asthma and several potent *leukotriene antagonists* are now in clinical trials. Results suggest that $LTD_4$ antagonists are relatively effective in blocking acute bronchoconstrictor challenges in asthmatic patients, but the future place of these drugs in the overall therapy of asthma is not yet established.

---

**Box 2.11 New treatments for asthma**

*New bronchodilators*

Long-acting inhaled $\beta$-agonists (e.g. salmeterol, formoterol)
Novel xanthine derivatives (e.g. enprofylline)
Selective muscarinic antagonists (under development)
Potassium channel activators (e.g. cromakalim)
Selective phosphodiesterase inhibitors

*New anti-inflammatory drugs*

More topical inhaled steroids (fluticasone, tipredane)
Mediator antagonists (leukotriene D4 antagonists such as ICI 204, 219)
Immunomodulators (inhaled cyclosporin, FK 506)
Modulators of neurogenic inflammation (substance P antagonists, peripherally acting opioids)
Cytokine inhibitors and antagonists (under development)

---

Several potent *PAF antagonists* and *thromboxane antagonists* are also being tested in asthma, but results are very disappointing and it is unlikely that these antagonists will be useful therapeutically.

Inhibition of enzymes involved in the synthetic pathway of lipid mediators are also under development. 5-lipoxygenase inhibitors which would block the formation of all leukotrienes and their immediate precursors may have an advantage over drugs which block a single receptor type. There is some preliminary evidence that they may be useful in asthma, but currently available compounds are not able to completely inhibit enzyme activity and more potent compounds are needed. Phospholipase $A_2$ is the enzyme which leads to the formation of arachidonic acid, which subsequently generates leukotrienes and prostaglandins, and of lyso-PAF, the precursor of PAF. Inhibition of PLA2 would thus block the formation of all lipid mediators and presumably be a valuable potential therapy in asthma. Unfortunately it has not proved possible to develop useful drugs in this category which are suitable for clinical use.

## Immunomodulators

Since altered mucosal immunity is fundamental to asthma, drugs which suppress the abnormal immune response may be useful in the treatment of chronic asthma. Indeed, corticosteroids may produce their effects by suppressing the abnormal immune response through inhibition of cytokine synthesis. In the future more specific drugs which block the synthesis or receptors of specific cytokines (such as the eosinophil specific cytokine interleukin-5) may be developed.

Drugs which inhibit T-lymphocyte function may also be developed in the future. Cyclosporin A, which is currently available, is too toxic to consider for general use, but other drugs with a similar effect (e.g. FK 506 and rapamycin) are under development. These drugs may be effective and less toxic via inhalation.

## FURTHER READING

Barnes P J 1989 A new approach to asthma therapy. New England Journal of Medicine 321: 1517–1527

Barnes P J 1992 New therapeutic approaches in asthma. British Medical Bulletin 48: 149–168

Barnes P J, Rodger I W, Thomson N C (eds) 1992 Asthma: basic mechanisms and clinical management 2nd edn. Academic Press, London.

British Thoracic Society 1993 Guidelines on the management of asthma. Thorax 48 (supplement): S1–S24

Hargreave F E, Dolovich J, Newhouse M T 1990 The assessment and treatment of asthma: a conference report. Journal of Allergy and Clinical Immunology 85: 1098–1111

Jenne J W, Murphy S (eds) 1987 Drug therapy for Asthma: Research and Clinical Practice. Dekker, New York

National Heart Lung and Blood Institute 1991 Guidelines for the diagnosis and management of asthma. Journal of Allergy and Clinical Immunology 88: 425–534

Warner J O et al 1989 Management of asthma: a consensus statement. Archive of Diseases of Childhood 64: 1065–1079

CHAPTER CONTENTS

**Introduction  49**
Pathophysiology and implications for therapy  49
Epidemiology  50
Clinical practice  50

**Pharmacotherapy in respiratory
failure  50**
Oxygen therapy  51
    Fixed performance devices  51
    Variable performance devices  51
    CPAP  51
    Long-term domiciliary oxygen therapy  51
    Transtracheal oxygen delivery  52
    Portable oxygen therapy  53
    Short-burst oxygen therapy  54
Bronchodilators  54
Vasodilators  54
Mucolytic agents  54
Respiratory stimulants  55
    Analeptics  55
    Methylxanthines  55
    Progestational hormones  56
    Carbonic anhydrase inhibitors  56
    Almitrine bismesylate  56
Carbonic anhydrase inhibition  56
Diuretics  57
Non invasive mechanical ventilation  57

**Respiratory muscle weakness  58**
Therapy  58
    Methylxanthines  58
    Sympathomimetic amines  59
    Digitalis  59
    Nutrition  59
    Nasal intermittent positive pressure ventilation  60

**Sleep apnoea  60**
Clinical presentation and diagnosis  61
General approach  61
    Upper airway obstruction  61
    Pharmacotherapy  61
    Nasal CPAP  61
    Tracheostomy  62

**Application of therapies In clinical
practice  62**
    Pure ventilatory failure  62
    Hypoxaemic respiratory failure  62
    Mixed ventilatory and hypoxaemic failure  62
    Obstructive sleep apnoea  64

**Summary  64**

# 3

# Respiratory failure

## INTRODUCTION

Type I respiratory failure may be defined as hypoxaemia resulting from any clinical condition leading to an arterial oxygen tension ($Pa_{O_2}$) of 8 kPa or less. Patients who have additionally an arterial carbon dioxide tension ($Pa_{CO_2}$) of 6.5 kPa or more are said to be in Type II failure (Box 3.1). The term cor pulmonale is used to define the association of hypoxaemic respiratory failure in association with right ventricular enlargement secondary to pulmonary hypertension and peripheral oedema. Patients with cor pulmonale have a poor clinical prognosis and over 60% are dead within 5 years of diagnosis.

## Pathophysiology and implications for therapy

Chronic hypoxaemia may result from a low inspired oxygen concentration ($FIO_2$); increased

---

**Box 3.1  Respiratory failure: classification**

*Type I*
Arterial oxygen tension ($Pa_{O_2}$) less than 60 mm Hg
(8 kPa) with normal carbon dioxide tensions ($Pa_{CO_2}$)

*Type II*
$Pa_{O_2}$ less than 60 mm Hg (8 kPa) and $Pa_{CO_2}$ above
50 mm Hg (6.7 kPa)

---

resistance to gas flow between the atmosphere and alveoli; impaired diffusion of oxygen across the alveolar capillary membrane, or respiratory muscle weakness. $Paco_2$ is dependent upon alveolar ventilation, $CO_2$ being more highly diffusible than oxygen. Therapeutic interventions are therefore aimed at reversing one or all of these pathophysiological mechanisms.

## Epidemiology

Deaths attributable to chronic obstructive pulmonary disease (COPD), the commonest cause of cor pulmonale, are falling in the UK from an estimated maximum of 30 000 per year in the 1950s and 1960s to a projected 7000 p.a. by the turn of the century. The improvement is largely attributable to the Clean Air Acts of the past 30 years and the gradual decline in cigarette smoking over the same period. Unfortunately, both environmental pollution and cigarette smoking are becoming increasingly common in the third world and cor pulmonale will be a major health concern for developing countries in the early part of the next century.

## Clinical practice

In clinical practice, the physiological abnormalities discussed above lead to three distinct patterns of respiratory disturbance (Table 3.1). Pure ventilatory failure, such as occurs following respiratory centre depression, results in a raised $Paco_2$ and low $Pao_2$; hypoxaemic respiratory failure (low $Pao_2$, low or normal $Paco_2$), which is seen in acute severe asthma or pneumonia; and a mixture of hypoxaemic and ventilatory disturbances leading to a low $Pao_2$ and raised $Paco_2$ (e.g. in chronic obstructive pulmonary disease, COPD). In the latter, chronic $CO_2$ retention usually results in chronic retention of bicarbonate leading to a compensated respiratory acidosis (unlike pure ventilatory failure).

Diagnosis depends upon eliciting a careful history (particularly of previous respiratory disease) and obtaining (in order) arterial gas analysis, a chest radiograph and culture of sputum and blood to exclude infection. Physical signs are often few and relatively non-specific (e.g. cyanosis, confusion). Simple spirometry to confirm or exclude airflow limitation can be useful. Chronic respiratory failure leads eventually to cor pulmonale.

## PHARMACOTHERAPY IN RESPIRATORY FAILURE

Drug therapy is aimed at correcting the physiological abnormalities associated with the condi-

**Table 3.1  Clinical patterns of respiratory failure**

*Pure ventilatory failure (raised $Paco_2$, low $Pao_2$)*
Respiratory centre depression (drugs, cerebrovascular accident)
Neurological impairment (Guillain-Barré syndrome, poliomyelitis, myasthenia gravis)
Alveolar hypoventilation (Pickwickian syndrome)

*Hypoxaemic failure (low $Pao_2$, low/normal $Paco_2$)*
Early stages of asthma attack
Massive pulmonary embolus
Emphysema
Pneumonia
Adult respiratory distress syndrome
Pulmonary oedema (left ventricular failure)

*Mixture of ventilatory and hypoxaemic failure (low $Pao_2$, high $Paco_2$)*
Chronic obstructive pulmonary disease (COPD)

**Table 3.2  Means of administering oxygen therapy**

| Device | Oxygen flow (l/min) | Oxygen concentration |
|---|---|---|
| Nasal cannulae | 2 | 29–35 |
|  | 4 | 32–39 |
| Hudson mask | 2 | 24–38 |
|  | 4 | 35–45 |
|  | 6 | 51–60 |
| MC mask | 2 | 28–50 |
|  | 4 | 41–70 |
|  | 6 | 53–74 |

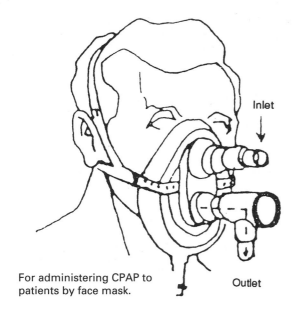

For administering CPAP to
patients by face mask.

**Fig. 3.1** Downs CPAP mask.

tions listed in Table 3.1. Therapeutic options
will be considered in turn.

## Oxygen therapy

Oxygen was established as a therapeutic agent
by J S Haldane in 1917. The breathing of oxy-
gen-enriched air was considered palliative to
damaged tissues as repair processes took place.
Its application in respiratory failure depends
upon the presence of absence of carbon dioxide
retention and is discussed in more detail below.
Oxygen can be administered in one of several
ways (Table 3.2):

### Fixed performance devices

These provide an inspired gas mixture of
known composition. Consequently, the $FIO_2$
does not vary in response to alterations in the
patient's pattern of respiration. This is the
principle behind the Ventimask.

### Variable performance devices

Oxygen is supplied at a flow rate less than the
patient's minute volume and the $FIO_2$ is deter-

mined by the interrelationship of these two factors. If the tidal volume varies from breath-to-
breath, the administered $FIO_2$ will also change.
Nasal cannulae, the Mary Catterall (MC) and
Hudson masks are all variable performance
devices.

### Continuous positive pressure ventilation (CPAP)

CPAP is useful in patients with a tendency
towards airway or pulmonary collapse at low
lung volumes. It diminishes work of breathing
and decreases hypoxaemia secondary to pulmonary oedema in patients with congestive
heart failure, traumatic lung injury or flail chest;
and is also useful in a variety of interstitial lung
diseases and infections. The resultant increase
in functional residual capacity (FRC) improves
ventilation–perfusion mismatch and arterial
oxygenation. Increased compliance reduces the
work of breathing. CPAP therefore reduces the
requirement for mechanical ventilation and an
increased $FIO_2$. It may be supplied using a tight-
ly fitting face mask (e.g. Downs Mask, Fig. 3.1)
and a flow generator operating from wall oxygen (Fig. 3.2). Gas is entrained such that flow
rates of up to 70–80 l/min are achieved ensuring that the airway pressure remains positive
relative to atmospheric even during inspiration
(Fig. 3.2).

### Long-term domiciliary oxygen therapy

Between acute exacerbations, patients with
Type II respiratory failure remain chronically
hypoxaemic and hypercapnic. Eventually, cor
pulmonale develops, with severe prognostic
implications. Long-term domiciliary oxygen
therapy provided at flow rates sufficient to raise
$Pao_2$ to at least 8 kPa for 15 or more hours a
day is the only treatment that has been shown
conclusively to improve survival. This was
demonstrated by two large-scale trials carried
out in the UK and USA in the late 1970s. In the
former, patients with severe hypoxaemic cor
pulmonale were randomly allocated to oxygen

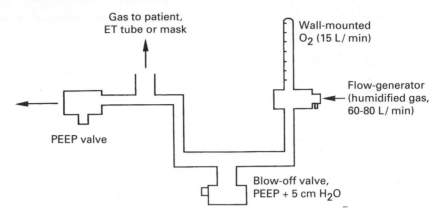

**Fig. 3.2** Typical circuit for the administration of continuous positive airways pressure (CPAP). Note gas flows in the region of 70–80 l/min are required to avoid airway pressure falling below atmospheric during inspiration.

provided via nasal cannulae at flow rates sufficient to raise $Pao_2$ to 8 kPa or more, usually 2 1/min) for 15 hours per day, or no oxygen. At the end of the study, a clear benefit in terms of mortality was demonstrated for those taking oxygen, amounting to a 50% reduction for males. The USA-based trial examined similar patients randomly allocated to 'continuous' (in practice some 19 hours per day) or 12 hours' oxygen therapy per day. After 19 months the mortality in the 12-hour group was almost double that of the 19-hour group and the trial was stopped (Fig. 3.3).

Thus, improvement seemed to depend upon the provision of at least 15 hours' oxygen per day, but was maintained long-term in a recent follow up of survivors from the original trial. Unfortunately, the changes in pulmonary vasculature in these patients seemed not to be reversed and elevated pulmonary vascular resistance, so characteristic of this condition (particularly on exercise), persists.

The early provision of long-term domiciliary oxygen therapy was costly and onerous as patients needed up to 13 cylinders per week, each of 48 cu ft, to achieve 15 hours' therapy per day. The development of special oxygen conserving devices built in to nasal cannulae was designed to overcome the former problem, but the advent of the oxygen concentrator to a cer-

tain extent obviated this problem. These are small, electrically driven machines capable of separating nitrogen from oxygen by a molecular 'sieve' and providing a stream of 100% oxygen at flow rates of up to 4 l/min. They can be prescribed by general practitioners, but studies of domiciliary oxygen provided in this manner have suggested that close supervision is needed. Thus, inadequate usage by patients in terms of the number of hours taken, the arterial gas tensions achieved and the reliability of the machines have all been documented. Furthermore, such therapy remains onerous for the patient, despite the use of lengths of tubing laid around the house to increase mobility, and a progressive reduction in the size and noise output of concentrators.

In the face of these difficulties, there has been increasing work considering the use of vasodilator therapy and combinations of oxygen therapy with respiratory stimulants in such patients, in order to reduce or obviate the requirement for oxygen provided for the majority of each day (see almitrine, Ch. 8 on pulmonary vascular disease).

### Transtracheal oxygen delivery

Transtracheal oxygen (TTO) therapy administered via a chronically implanted catheter is a

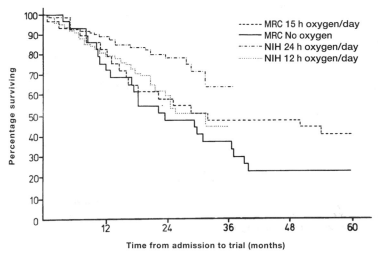

**Fig. 3.3** Effects of long-term domiciliary oxygen therapy on mortality (NOTT and MRC trials).

practice that has gained much momentum in the USA in recent years, but remains relatively unpopular in Europe. In addition to oxygen conservation (a lower flow is required to produce the same $Pao_2$ achieved by higher flow rates delivered via nasal cannulae), advocates of this approach point out that compliance may be improved and the nasal and auricular irritation frequently experienced using cannulae is obviated. Studies have shown that the catheters need be replaced only every 2 months. Complications include sputum plugging, infection and minor haemoptyses. Probably the only patients in whom this approach offers significant advantages are those with hypoxaemia refractory to oxygen delivered via nasal prongs at the highest flow rate of a concentrator, or those wishing to spend a good deal of time away from home and wishing to extend considerably the duration of a portable system.

### Portable oxygen therapy

Portable oxygen has been advocated for those patients with severe respiratory insufficiency, to increase exercise performance and decrease dyspnoea. The theoretical basis for this assumption is clear, but until the early 1980s the benefits likely to accrue from this approach were difficult to quantify. Two important developments in respiratory physiology made the evaluation of oxygen therapy in these circumstances possible. Oxygen was found to improve treadmill performance in patients with COPD as early as 1955, but the advent of the 12-minute walking test for assessing disability in such patients greatly simplified matters. However, the objective assessment of breathlessness, a sensation probably due to a central assimilation of physiological (i.e. altered perception of control of respiration and disturbed recognition of added resistive and elastic loads) and psychological factors proved difficult. The advent of the visual analogue scale (VAS) of breathlessness, whereby patients are asked to grade their breathlessness by marking a point on a 100 mm line labelled at the extremes 'none' and 'severe', has assisted such studies enormously. VAS has evolved into an accurate and reproducible measurement of what was previously considered a purely subjective sensation.

Work carried out in the early 1980s using these techniques in patients with severe COPD suggested that the benefit patients can attain from carrying (or wheeling) a portable supply of oxygen (e.g. Portagen system, weighing 2 kg, sufficient for up to 40 min at 2 l/min via nasal prongs) could be up to 15% increase in distance walked. Nevertheless, due to the severe nature of disease, this might amount to only 20–30 yards in absolute distance walked. However, more significantly in both the major studies performed, a clear improvement in distressing dyspnoea was observed, representing an obvious therapeutic benefit. Interestingly, breathlessness and simple exercise capacity may respond independently to oxygen. It seems clear, however, in view of the highly emotive nature of the therapy, that the use of portable oxygen needs to be carefully evaluated in individual patients in a placebo-controlled fashion.

### Short-burst oxygen therapy

Breathlessness and reduced exercise tolerance are the major complaints of patients suffering from chronic airflow limitation. As has been seen, the prescription of oxygen for such patients is haphazard. Thus, studies have shown that although oxygen is prescribed for the relief of hypoxaemia, it is taken by patients overwhelmingly for the relief of breathlessness. As such studies have also demonstrated that the therapy is taken in the vast majority of cases for periods between a few minutes and half an hour, it is clearly unlikely to substantially reverse hypoxaemia. Physicians have therefore tended to discount the value of oxygen taken in this manner, regarding improvements in subjective sensations such as breathlessness as a placebo response to a highly emotive treatment.

Nevertheless, a number of recent studies have shown this opinion to be unfounded. Using standardised exercise tests and the VAS in placebo-controlled trials, it has been demonstrated that a number of patients with severe COPD achieve more rapid diminution in breathlessness following exercise breathing oxygen than air. Physiological recovery, as assessed by resolution of tachycardia and respiratory rate, are unaffected. As before, it is clear that variation between individuals is great and placebo-controlled trials need to be performed in each case to assess those likely to achieve the greatest benefit.

## Bronchodilators

The applications of bronchodilator therapy in patients with obstructive airflow limitation are discussed in Chapter 2.

## Vasodilators

The use of pulmonary vasodilators in cor pulmonale is discussed in more detail in Chapter 3.

## Mucolytic agents

Much research has been devoted to improving bronchopulmonary clearance of secretions in Type II respiratory failure and a number of pharmacological agents have been produced to achieve this end with varying results (Box 3.2). Mucociliary function is markedly impaired in patients with COPD and gravity and cough may be the most effective stimuli to bronchial clearance. Of the agents listed in Box 3.2, N-acetylcysteine (NAC) is probably the most effective. Claims have been made following large-scale European trials that NAC may reduce the frequency and severity of infective exacerbations in COPD, but mucolytic agents are rarely used in the UK. Trials during acute exacerbations have been less conclusive, partic-

---

**Box 3.2  Pharmacological agents designed to facilitate bronchopulmonary clearance of secretions**

Saturated solution of potassium iodide
Ammonium chloride
Glyceryl guaiacolate
Bromhexine
S-carboxymethylcysteine
N-acetylcysteine
Water/aerosols/ultrasonic nebulisation
Vibratory chest percussion

ularly as the drug is hypertonic when administered by aerosol and irritating, leading to mucosal oedema after prolonged use. Oral preparations may be more effective and may have a protective effect against smoke-induced injury and other air pollutants

## Respiratory stimulants

During acute exacerbations of COPD, increases in $FIO_2$ may be needed to achieve an adequate $Pao_2$, but may cause an acute rise in $Paco_2$, probably resulting from a reduction in hypoxic drive and an acquired insensitivity to carbon dioxide. In theory, respiratory stimulants would be an attractive means of reducing the requirement for oxygen therapy during periods of stability and might be expected to prevent this rise in $PaCO_2$ during exacerbations. Respiratory stimulants can be broadly classified as shown in Box 3.3.

### Analeptics

Central nervous system stimulants that can be considered analeptics include nikethamide and doxepram. Both drugs increase arousal and the

---

**Box 3.3  Classification of respiratory stimulants**

*Analeptics*
Nikethamide
Doxepram

*Methylxanthines*
Theophylline

*Hormones*
Medroxyprogesterone

*Tricyclic antidepressant*
Protriptyline

*Carbonic anhydrase inhibitors*
Actetazolamide

*Triazine derivative*
Almitrine bismesylate

---

**Box 3.4   Dose regimen for doxepram**

In acute respiratory failure the following has been shown to result in a steady state plasma concentration of drug:

| | |
|---|---|
| 0–15 min | 4.0 mg/min |
| 15–30 min | 3.0 mg/min |
| 30–60 min | 2.0 mg/min |
| 60 min plus | 1.5 mg/min |

---

response to sensory stimulation and stimulate respiration, probably by directly increasing CNS excitation at all levels of the brain and spinal cord. Doxepram has a direct stimulatory effect on the carotid chemoreceptors at low doses. Both may therefore have a role in increasing arousal following general anaesthesia. Doxepram is administered intravenously (usually as doxepram hydrochloride 2 mg/ml in 500 ml 5% dextrose; dose regimen shown in Box 3.4), is rapidly cleared from the circulation (principally by liver metabolism) and is a more potent and specific respiratory stimulant than nikethamide (2–5 ml, 0.5–1.25 mg), producing less generalised stimulation and with a higher threshold for inducing grand mal convulsions. Doxepram also influences respiratory timing through vagal or medullary-pontine pathways, increasing mean inspiratory flow rate and occlusion pressure, tidal volume and frequency. The effects of doxepram are delayed or blunted by concurrent oxygen administration, but at levels of 1.6–3.0 µg/ml, it increases the ventilatory responses to both hypoxia and hypercapnia in the absence of changes in oxygen consumption or $CO_2$ production. Doxepram is also effective in alleviating laryngeal spasm after tracheal intubation.

### Methylxanthines

Theophylline and caffeine are potent central nervous system stimulants causing nervousness, insomnia and tremors. Theophylline increases respiratory activity by a direct effect on brain-stem respiratory centres causing increases in resting ventilation in a dose-dependent fashion; increasing the ventilatory response to hypoxia and raising the volume of ventilation at any given $Paco_2$ during hypercapnia. These effects are particularly apparent in infancy and the methylxanthines are probably most widely used in the management of idiopathic apnoea of prematurity. The ability of theophylline to improve the contractility of the respiratory muscles is discussed below.

### Progestational hormones

Progestational agents have been shown to stimulate respiration in both normal subjects and those with respiratory disorders through unknown mechanisms. Changes in minute ventilation are mediated through increased tidal volume. The effects of medroxyprogesterone during sleep have been inconsistent and the possibility of complications following long-term use have not been fully evaluated.

### Carbonic anhydrase inhibitors

(See below).

### Tricyclic antidepressants

Protriptylline, a non-sedating tricyclic antidepressant agent, has been used to improve the drowsiness and cataplexy associated with narcolepsy, resulting in fewer and shorter periods of apnoea. The use of protryptilline starting at 10 mg b.d. and adjusting the dose according to clinical effect and side-effects has also been very successful in patients with sleep-disordered breathing. Nevertheless, variations in therapeutic response have been considerable and severe anti-cholinergic side-effects (dry mouth, sexual impotence, constipation and urinary hesitancy) are reported in up to 50% of patients. The drug works by reducing the period spent in rapid eye movement (REM) sleep, the period most associated with sleep apnoea, although it actually has few effects on the polysomnograph. In mild obstructive sleep-disordered breathing its

effects are attributed to the selective activation of motor neurons to the upper airway muscles.

### Almitrine bismesylate

Almitrine bismesylate, a triazine derivative, is a recently-developed oral respiratory stimulant that differs from previous respiratory agonists by acting on peripheral chemoreceptors, principally the carotid body, to increase tidal volume. In clinical trials in patients with COPD, almitrine has been shown to increase $Pao_2$ by 0.5–1.2 kPa and reduce $Paco_2$ by up to 1.0 kPa. The drug seems to be generally well tolerated, the most frequent complaints being increased breathlessness, nausea and non-specific malaise all of which are related to drug concentrations. Early regimens (100 mg b.d.) tended to lead to drug accumulation in patients with COPD, particularly after several months' administration, with half-lives of up to 1–3 weeks being reported. Delayed clearance of drug may also occur in patients with cirrhosis. The long half-life may be due to the very large volume of distribution of the drug or low plasma clearance. Current thinking suggests that 50 mg b.d. or even once daily may be sufficient for a maximal response. Almitrine has been reported to cause breathlessness in normal subjects and in patients with COPD, with an increased incidence at higher drug concentrations; other trials, however, have reported a reduction in dyspnoea scores. The drug is still undergoing trials in the UK.

Although the use of respiratory stimulants may appear attractive, thus far their clinical application (except in specific circumstances) has been associated with little evidence of proven benefit and many undesirable side-effects.

## Carbonic anhydrase inhibition

Patients with ventilatory/hypoxaemic respiratory failure usually present with a respiratory acidosis and high plasma bicarbonate, reflecting a partial metabolic compensation for their chronic $CO_2$ retention. Consequently, following correction of their hypoxaemia and reduction of

$Paco_2$, their high levels of bicarbonate persist, at least in the short term. Even if $Paco_2$ can be normalised, bicarbonate levels frequently remain high for many days, buffering $CO_2$ that is retained by the patient and further inhibiting respiratory drive. The respiratory centre can be 're-set' to respond to hypercarbia if renal excretion of bicarbonate is promoted through the use of acetazolamide (250–500 mg/d for 3–5 d). The drug increases cerebral blood flow, decreases CSF bicarbonate and increases the responsiveness of the respiratory centre. Furthermore, the mild non-respiratory acidaemia induced by acetazolamide may provide a useful pathway to increased oxygenation during hypoxia by shifting the oxyhaemoglobin dissociation curve, facilitating oxygen release and increasing ventilation, in much the same way as it does when being used for the treatment of acute mountain sickness.

## Diuretics

There is considerable evidence that patients with exacerbations of COPD have an impaired ability to excrete a salt and water load, thus contributing to the build up of peripheral oedema.

Furthermore, acute hypoxaemia almost certainly causes a re-distribution of intra-renal blood flow and diuretics are frequently ineffective in the absence of oxygen therapy. More over, if the patient is concomitantly taking steroids and $\beta_2$-agonists, non-potassium sparing diuretics can lead to severe potassium depletion which can exacerbate the tendency towards dysrhythmias (already high in hypoxaemic patients), thereby intensifying muscular weakness and debility. Combination therapy with frusemide (40 mg) and amiloride (5 mg) (Frumil, 1–2 tablets daily) is usually satisfactory. The competitive aldosterone antagonist spironolactone (initially 3 mg/kg body weight, increasing to 400 mg/d) was considered by many to be the drug of choice in severe cor pulmonale, but is contraindicated in patients with renal impairment. Long-term use has also been discouraged since the emergence of reports of carcinogenicity in experimental animals.

It is probably reasonable to restrict the use of diuretics to patients with marked hepatic engorgement or in whom there is evidence of left ventricular failure. There is no therapeutic merit in the rapid reduction of peripheral oedema per se, which will probably occur spontaneously with improved oxygenation.

## Non-invasive mechanical ventilation

The majority of cases with reversible disease leading to pure ventilatory failure will need mechanical ventilatory support supplied in the conventional fashion via a cuffed endotracheal tube. Nevertheless, non-invasive means of supplying ventilatory support have been available through the application of intermittent negative pressure (INPV) to the chest wall (as in the 'tank' ventilator or iron lung). The cuirass shell, pneumosuit and Tunicliffe jacket are portable forms of negative pressure equipment, but require bulky pumps to create intermittent sub-atmospheric pressure around the thorax. INPV is unwieldy and unsuitable for use by patients with high thoracic impedance and/or intrinsic pulmonary disease, such as in COPD. For this patient population, nasal intermittent positive pressure ventilation (NIPPV) administered via a tightly-fitting mask held around the nose, has proved very successful. Both volume- and pressure-cycled machines are used. The former delivers a stable tidal volume in the face of changing pulmonary characteristics, such as compliance; but the latter can counteract leaks more effectively even though it cannot adapt to variations in lung compliance and airways resistance. Using NIPPV, patients with a variety of chronic pathologies can be 'tided over' an episode of acute respiratory failure without resorting to intubation. This comparatively recent development is proving particularly use-

---

**Box 3.5  Respiratory muscle weakness: drugs and interventions**

*Pharmacotherapy*

| | |
|---|---|
| Methylxanthines: | theophylline |
| | caffeine |
| Sympathomimetic amines: | salbutamol |
| | terbutaline |
| | dopamine |

Digitalis

*Nutrition*

Patients < 90% of ideal body weight
Calorific intake < 40% above baseline
Composition probably unimportant
Weight gain and maintenance of increased calorie intake essential

*Nasal positive pressure ventilation*

Unlikely to be successful as substitute for conventional mechanical ventilation in patients unable to tolerate spontaneous breathing for < 20–25 min.

---

ful in patients with COPD and/or respiratory muscle weakness (see below). Modified devices are suitable for the management of patients with sleep apnoea (see below).

## RESPIRATORY MUSCLE WEAKNESS

Evidence accumulated in recent years suggests that respiratory muscle weakness contributes significantly to the limitation in exercise capacity, dyspnoea and respiratory failure associated with a number of pulmonary and non-pulmonary pathologies. Respiratory muscle fatigue may result from pathology within the central nervous system, a failure of neuromuscular transmission or impaired muscle contractility. There is considerable controversy regarding the point at which the system is most vulnerable. Furthermore, only recently has it been recognised that the muscles may be unable to generate the appropriate force despite an adequate neural drive. This last issue is clearly critical in determining the part played by so-called air

pump dysfunction in the genesis of dyspnoea in patients with COPD.

## Therapy

The investigation of respiratory muscle weakness requires considerable expertise in assessing such parameters as phrenic nerve conduction, trans-diaphragmatic pressure changes and EMGs. Therapeutic interventions are still under evaluation. They include mechanical support using non-invasive positive pressure ventilation, attention to feeding and nutrition and a number of drugs, particularly the methylxanthines and sympathetic amines (Box 3.5).

### Methylxanthines

Caffeine and theophylline have long been known to increase the force generated by isolated muscle strips to which electrical stimulation is applied in vitro. Thus, diaphragmatic contractility is increased in dogs with high-dose theophylline (sufficient to produce a plasma concentration of around 100 mg/l). In early studies performed in normal human subjects aminophylline (plasma concentration 13± 0.9 mg/l), unlike caffeine, was found to increase transdiaphragmatic contractility as assessed by occluded maximal inspiratory threshold loading and to decrease the sense of effort during loaded breathing.

Unfortunately, measuring diaphragmatic force frequency curves is technically difficult. Despite using other muscle groups and repeating studies in normal individuals and patients with chronic respiratory insufficiency, most investigations have yielded mixed or negative results. On the basis of current evidence it seems that aminophylline has no effect on skeletal muscle strength or fatigability and does not increase respiratory muscle strength when full activation of the respiratory muscles is achieved. Diaphragmatic endurance is not improved by aminophylline, but the drug may increase the force of a submaximal contraction in both the fresh and fatigued states in a minor (< 20% augmentation) fashion.

## Sympathomimetic amines

Sympathomimetic amines have been known for some time to increase twitch amplitude and duration, thereby potentiating tension in fast twitch muscle in vitro. Furthermore, terbutaline has been shown to increase trans-diaphragmatic pressure generation during both low and high frequency electrical stimulation in dog respiratory muscle in both the fresh and fatigued state. However, high dose (4 mg t.d.s.) salbutamol has been shown to have no significant effect on diaphragmatic strength or endurance in normal human subjects in either the fresh or fatigued state. There are two possible explanations for such disappointing results. The human diaphragm has relatively few fast twitch fibres compared with dogs, and in vitro it is the contractility of these fibres that is increased by $\beta_2$-agonists. Alternatively, it is possible that some amines (e.g. dopamine) increase diaphragmatic contractility in experimental preparations through changes in blood flow rather than via a direct action on diaphragmatic contractility. Oral terbutaline has no significant effects on either maximal inspiratory pressure or maximal trans-diaphragmatic pressure in patients with COPD.

In summary, $\beta_2$-agonists appear to have little effect on diaphragmatic strength or endurance in humans. Whether they can alter the force–frequency curve of the fatigued diaphragm in humans as they do in animals remains to be seen. Initial studies considering the effects of dopamine on respiratory muscle function in the critically ill patient are of sufficient interest to warrant further investigation.

## Digitalis

In vitro data have suggested that digoxin in doses sufficient to induce therapeutic plasma concentrations (1–2 ng/ml) does not influence diaphragmatic contractility in vitro. However, in large animals in vivo digoxin may increase contractility as assessed for force–frequency curves. In a single study in patients in the fresh non-fatigued state, the drug also increased trans-diaphragmatic twitch pressure.

In conclusion, although there is no drug presently available that unambiguously improves the performance of the respiratory pump, there are sufficient encouraging preliminary studies to suggest that effective therapeutic intervention in this area may not be far away.

## Nutrition

Malnutrition is an important clinical problem in a sub-population of patients with COPD. In a recent study carried out in the USA, nearly 25% of patients with stable COPD weighed less than 90% of their ideal body weight. It appears that the prevalence of malnutrition increases with the severity of airflow limitation and approaches or even exceeds 50% in investigations examining patients admitted to hospital for exacerbations of their condition. Reduced respiratory muscle mass and function as well as increased susceptibility to infection are important consequences of malnutrition which in themselves may also contribute substantially to mortality in this group of patients.

The degree to which nutritional support is necessary depends on the perception as to whether the problem can be attributed to reduced energy intake or increased energy expenditure. Indirect calorimetry suggests that patients with stable COPD have a 10–20% increase in resting energy expenditure, a feature attributed to the increased work of breathing. However total energy expenditure may be normal due to reduced physical activity consequent upon respiratory disability. It seems likely that weight loss is therefore a primary result of inadequate energy intake in relation to metabolic requirements.

In most studies, weight gain in patients with severe COPD can only be achieved by substantially increasing energy intake (greater than 30% above basal) and improvements in muscle function and exercise tolerance appear to be dependent upon patients actually gaining weight. Thus, in one series a mean weight gain of 4.2 kg achieved by increasing dietary intake by 48% above baseline levels over a 3-month period led to an increase in maximal respiratory muscle pressures and handgrip, and sternomastoid strength; together with a decrease in sternomastoid muscle fatigability. The control group saw no such improvements. In a second study, nasogastric feeding for 16 d, which increased energy intake by 75% above baseline caused a 2.4 kg increase in body weight and improved both respiratory muscle strength and endurance. No change in weight or muscle performance was observed in patients whose incremental energy intake was smaller, or in the control group. Unfortunately it seems possible that such gains are transitory if weight is lost when patients return to their usual diet.

Patients with COPD tend to tolerate carbohydrates without difficulty and although lower $CO_2$ production is associated with fat intake (RQ=0.7 cf carbohydrate RQ=1.0), most patients with COPD appear to tolerate carbohydrates without difficulty. Thus, in one study both normocapnic and hypercapnic patients maintained a constant $Paco_2$ after a 920 Kcal carbohydrate load. Low carbohydrate, high-fat formula feeds do not therefore seem to be necessary for nutritional support in patients with stable disease.

The best means of administrating nutritional support is also a matter for debate. Nocturnal supplemental feeding via a nasogastric tube has been used and proved to be effective in patients, but when oral supplements are used they need to be given at the end of or between meals such that the usual dietary intake is not impaired. Close monitoring and counselling is necessary if energy intake is to be maintained. Dedicated and specialised personnel are almost certainly necessary for such a programme to succeed.

Encouraging dietary supplements therefore seems to be appropriate in patients with stable COPD who are less than 90% of their stable body weight. The best way of achieving this in terms of administration of extra nutrition, the composition of the nutrition and the effect on mortality and morbidity are still unclear.

### Nasal intermittent positive pressure ventilation

NIPPV (see above) has also been used with success in weaning patients with respiratory muscle weakness from conventional mechanical ventilation and providing nocturnal support. There is some evidence for a training effect following prolonged NIPPV, in that when support is removed after 6 months' therapy resting arterial gas tensions are improved when compared with pre-NIPPV levels. However, initial evidence suggests that this is not due to a training or resting effect of the device, in that formal tests of respiratory muscle strength remain unaltered. Removing the patient dependent upon conventional mechanical ventilation administered via a cuffed ET or tracheostomy tube to NIPPV is a complex and potentially dangerous procedure, although the results can be gratifying. It is unlikely to be successful in subjects unable to tolerate spontaneous, unassisted ventilation for less than 20–25 minutes.

## SLEEP APNOEA

Sleep apnoea implies the cessation of breathing during sleep and is defined as cessation of airflow at the mouth and nose for a period of more than 10 seconds. Sleep apnoea syndrome (SAS) is present when the number of such episodes exceed 5–8 per hour. Apnoea is usually quantified as the number of apnoea episodes per hour of sleep (apnoea index) and can be subclassified into three types. Central sleep apnoea occurs due to failure of central respiratory drive and obstructive apnoea through obstruction of the upper airway resulting in cessation of airflow at the nose and mouth, although respiratory movements continue and even increase in intensity. In many patients both forms co-exist, usually with one form dominant.

# Clinical presentation and diagnosis

Significant sleep apnoea leads to snoring, fragmented and unsatisfactory sleep, insomnia, enuresis and hypnagogic hallucinations when sleep is attempted. Daytime somnolence, intellectual deterioration, headaches, memory impairment and loss of libido are also common complaints (Box 3.6). Recognition of symptoms such as these is important, but only as an indication that a simple screening test is advisable. The overnight recording of oxygen saturation ($Sao_2$) using a pulse oximeter will establish the presence or absence of significant falls in $Sao_2$ (defined as $> 4\%$). Transcutaneous electrodes are less reliable in adults. Episodic desaturation may be associated with syndromes other than apnoea or hypopnoea, but its absence makes sleep apnoea unlikely. When the diagnosis is suspected on the basis of history or screening tests, the patient should be referred to a centre with the facilities to measure $Sao_2$, thoracic or abdominal muscle movement, airflow at the nose and mouth and heart rate. Many laboratories also record transcutaneous $CO_2$ EEG, submental EMG and eye movements.

---

**Box 3.6  Clinical presentation in sleep apnoea**

| | |
|---|---|
| Common: | Excessive daytime somnolence |
| | Snoring or apnoea |
| | Obesity |
| Less common: | Nocturnal headache |
| | Enuresis |
| | Impotence psychiatric disorder |
| | Incidental polycythaemia, |
| |   respiratory failure |
| | In association with |
| |   hypothyroidism, acromegaly |

---

A full ENT assessment is necessary to exclude narrowing of the nasopharynx, usually associated with the obese patient and those with receding jaw, macroglossia, large tonsils or pendulous uvula. Nasal obstruction through polyps, rhinitis or displaced septum can also produce obstructive or central sleep apnoea.

# General approach

Dietary control of weight is extremely important in patients with sleep apnoea and may be successful in abolishing the syndrome altogether. Abstinence of alcohol before bedtime is similarly vital. Sedative or hypnotic agents should be avoided. If these measures are unsuccessful in abolishing the presenting symptoms (Box 3.6), admission for diagnostic sleep study is needed.

## Upper airway obstruction

If nasal obstruction is detected, anatomic abnormalities such as deviated nasal septum, narrowed nasal airway secondary to inflammation or chronic rhinitis may require appropriate therapy. Enlarged tonsils and adenoids may need to be removed. Micrognathia, retrognathia or other skeletal abnormalities may require evaluation by an ENT or oral surgeon. Uvulopharyngopalatoplasty (UPPP) is a surgical procedure designed to reduce the redundancy in the soft tissues of the palate and nasopharynx. Results are variable. Selecting those patients likely to benefit from this operation is also difficult. Dynamic endoscopic assessment of the upper airway while patients undertake valsalva and Muller's manoeuvres has been advocated. Complications to the surgery include obstruction of the upper airway in the post-operative period, bleeding and sore throat which can lead to disability lasting several weeks. Long-term complications include nasal regurgitation and difficulty in phonation.

## Pharmacotherapy

Patients with sleep apnoea with hypo-ventilation when awake (associated with elevated $Paco_2$ greater than 6.5 kPa) and an $FE_1$ greater than 1 l should be treated with medroxyprogesterone acetate (60 mg daily). The therapy is less successful in obese patients with sleep apnoea who have no hypo-ventilation when awake. In patients with obesity and mild to moderate obstructive apnoea protriptyline (10 mg b.d. adjusted upwards or downwards dependent upon clinical response) is indicated. Unpleasant side-effects may preclude the use of this drug (see above).

### Nasal CPAP

Nasal CPAP is used in the vast majority of patients with obstructive sleep apnoea to splint the upper airway open. This is administered via a tight fitting facemask and new commercially available systems are relatively well-designed and quiet. The level of CPAP required depends upon the results of sleep studies and data obtained at all sleep stages. In the majority of patients 7.5–12.5 cm $H_2O$ is adequate to maintain satisfactory oxygenation. Low pressure is required in thin patients with retrognathia but obese patients may require pressures in the range 15-20 cm $H_2O$. CPAP should be distinguished from NIPPV, which actually augments the patient's spontaneous minute volume. With CPAP, airway pressure is held above atmospheric throughout the respiratory cycle and the rate and volume of gas flow to the lungs is determined by the patient.

### Tracheostomy

If pharmacotherapy and CPAP are unsuccessful and the patient is unsuitable or unwilling to undertake surgery the permanent tracheostomy remains a therapeutic option. This is a highly effective form of therapy and with the use of a fenestrated tube the patient can be restored to a relatively normal existence. The serious complication rate appears to be low in the long term and patient acceptance high. Again, this is aggressive therapy more commonly employed in the USA than Europe.

## APPLICATION OF THERAPIES IN CLINICAL PRACTICE

A careful history and physical examination together with the following urgent investiga-tions should define the pattern of respiratory failure, thereby providing pointers towards the underlying diagnosis (Table 3.1) and appropriate management:

1. Arterial gas analysis
2. Chest radiograph
3. Sputum and blood cultures
4. Blood count; urea, electrolytes, glucose; liver function tests.

Immediate management is then determined by the underlying disease process. In many cases where respiratory failure is entirely consequent upon pathology involving a second organ system (e.g. left ventricular failure) pulmonary support (e.g. oxygen) should be provided until directed therapies (e.g. diuretics, inotropes) are effective. Management protocols provided here are therefore appropriate only for patients with 'primary' respiratory failure.

## Pure ventilatory failure

The combination of hypoxaemia and hypercapnia is usually a consequence of respiratory muscle weakness or respiratory centre depression by drugs, producing alveolar hypoventilation. In the absence of reversible pathology, where mechanical ventilation via a cuffed endotracheal tube is appropriate, nasal intermittent positive pressure ventilation is the treatment of choice.

## Hypoxaemic respiratory failure

'Pure' emphysema, asthma in the initial stages of an attack (see Ch. 2), pneumonia (see Ch. 4), fibrosing alveolitis or ARDS (see Ch. 8) present in this fashion. A combination of bronchodilator therapies, antibiotics and steroids should therefore be applied as appropriate. High inspired oxygen concentrations, applied in one of the ways described above, should be used to alleviate hypoxaemia whilst the underlying condition (e.g. bronchospasm, pulmonary oedema) is reversed. In such cases, either a Venturi device or nasal prongs will correct hypoxaemia without causing significant $CO_2$ retention. The effica-

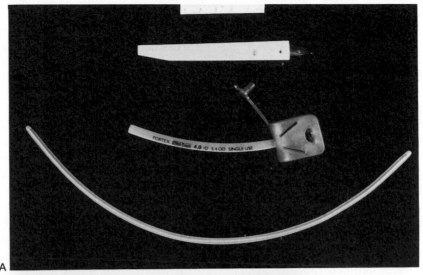

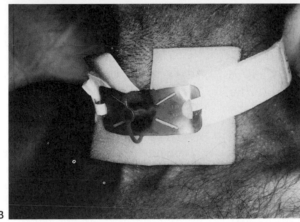

**Fig. 3.4**
Minitracheostomy:
(A) Contents of pre
packed 'kit'. (B)
Minitracheostomy in
place.

cy of nasal prongs in these circumstances is established. Even mouthbreathers effectively entrain oxygen into the nasopharynx and the device is more comfortable to use than a mask for prolonged periods.

## Mixed ventilatory and hypoxaemic failure

Acute exacerbations of chronic obstructive lung disease, leading to a low $Pao_2$ and high $Paco_2$ are the commonest cause of this pattern of respiratory insufficiency. The main aim of therapy is to increase intracellular $O_2$, whilst avoiding hyper-

capnia and treating any exacerbating factors such as infection. Thus, antibiotics and energetic attempts to remove secretions (by physiotherapy) are required. Nasotracheal suction (if necessary via a nasopharyngeal airway or minitracheostomy (Fig. 3.4) should be instigated. The latter is highly effective in assisting physiotherapy and may prevent recourse to intubation. Salbutamol (5 ml mixed with 3 ml 0.9% saline) should be given by nebuliser or IPPV up to 4 times daily. Aminophylline v (5 mg/kg initially and then 0.5 mg/h) should be administered, but plasma levels and drug interactions need to be carefully monitored. Steroids (hydrocortisone

200 mg/6 h) can also be given, although their efficacy in chronic airflow limitation is a matter of debate. Controlled, low flow oxygen therapy is required. The majority of patients with this type of respiratory failure have COPD and eventually develop a low respiratory sensitivity to $CO_2$. Their main chemical stimulus to breathing therefore becomes hypoxaemia sensed at peripheral chemoreceptors. If this drive is reduced through the administration of oxygen, hypoventilation occurs. These patients show a good correlation between the respiratory response to oxygen and resting $Paco_2$ when the patient is breathing air: that is the lower the $CO_2$ sensitivity the higher the resting $CO_2$. The use of oxygen in these circumstances requires special care if $CO_2$ retention is to be avoided. Respiratory stimulants are theoretically attractive, particularly if they could be used in combination with oxygen therapy, but have proved disappointing. Only doxepram is indicated (Box 3.4) if drug-induced CNS/respiratory drive suppression is suspected. The precise means of oxygen administration is also important. The 'Ventimask' (0.24 $FIO_2$, see above) should be used initially, increasing to 0.28 if the $Pao_2$ does not rise to at least 8.0 kPa. The use of nasal cannulae in these circumstances is a matter of some debate. Nasal stimulation may alter the pattern of respiration, thereby increasing alveolar ventilation and reducing $Paco_2$, but more frequently the delivered $FIO_2$ rises progressively as hypoxic respiratory drive is alleviated and the proportion of each tidal breath composed of oxygen increases, increasing the tendency towards hypercapnia. Pulse oximetry and the frequent assessment of arterial gas tensions is mandatory in these circumstances.

## Obstructive sleep apnoea

### Patients with upper airway obstruction

*General.* If the patient is found to have obstructive sleep apnoea the appropriate urgent therapy is nasal CPAP. If the patient has hypoventilation without episodes of apnoea, administration of medroxyprogesterone (60 mg daily) with monitoring until there is a response is indicated. In patients with hypercapnia treated with CPAP or medroxyprogesterone the reduction in arterial $CO_2$ tension may be rapid and cause serious alkalosis. In these circumstances blood bicarbonate concentrations are substantially above normal and the use of acetazolamide in these circumstances can be useful to maintain pH in the physiological range (see above). This drug also causes potassium loss and supplements may be required. The response to medroxyprogesterone is unpredictable and up to 2 weeks of continuous therapy may be required before response can be detected or refuted.

Phlebotomy to reduce polycythemia has been advocated when the haematocrit is in excess of 55%, particularly if the patient has neurological complaints. This approach is more commonly advocated in the USA than in the UK. The treatment of obstructive sleep apnoea involves attention to any underlying medical problems, weight reduction and avoidance of sedatives and alcohol. These simple measures are effective in many patients with mild or moderate symptoms.

The most effective medical therapeutic agents are the tricyclic anti-depressants. Protryptilline 5–30 mg daily alters the sleep state by reducing rapid eye movement (REM) sleep and may increase the tone of the upper airway muscles. The long-term benefit is variable and some patients deteriorate after a good initial response. Medroxyprogesterone has been of value in some patients with OSA, but the hormonal side-effects are frequently unacceptable. Other drugs such as theophylline and almitrine confer no benefit.

*Surgical.* Detailed discussion of surgical interventions are beyond the scope of this book and apply principally to the obstructive syndrome. Uvulopalatopharyngoplasty (UVPPP) increases the size of the oropharyngeal lumen by excising redundant tissue and usually improves snoring, although its effect on nocturnal desaturation is less predictable.

## SUMMARY

Patients in respiratory failure may be hypoxaemic due to a low inspired oxygen concentration ($FIO_2$); may suffer from obstruction to, or increased resistance to gas flow between the atmosphere and alveoli; or may have impaired diffusion of oxygen across the alveolar capillary membrane, or respiratory muscle weakness. They may also suffer from hypercapnia due to alveolar hypoventilation. In this chapter, the use of oxygen, respiratory stimulants and agents designed to obviate sleep apnoea and improve respiratory muscle function have been discussed.

FURTHER READING

Evans T W, Tweney J, Waterhouse J C, Nichol J, Suggett A J, Howard P 1990 Almitrine bismesylate and oxygen therapy in hypoxic cor pulmonale. Thorax 45: 16–21

Fitting J W 1992 Nutritional support in chronic obstructive lung disease. Thorax 47: 141–142

Mador M Jeffrey 1990 Pharmacotherapy of the respiratory muscles. In: Tobin M (ed) Problems in respiratory care: vol. 13, No. 3: The respiratory muscles. Lippincott, USA

Moxham J (ed) 1991 Assisted ventilation. British Medical Journal

**Introduction   67**

**Antibiotics used in respiratory infections   67**
Penicillins   68
Cephalosporins   69
Aminoglycosides   69
Macrolides   69
Co-trimoxazole   70
Tetracyclines   70
Quinolones   70
New ß-lactams   71
Vancomycin   71
Clindamycin   71

**Upper respiratory tract infections   71**
Rhinitis   72
Sinusitis   72
Pharyngitis   73
Laryngotracheitis and epiglottitis   73
Otitis media   73

**Lower respiratory tract infections   73**
Pneumonias   73
Clinical approach to pneumonia   74
   Community-acquired pneumonia   74
   Hospital-acquired pneumonia   75
   Aspiration pneumonia   75
   Immunocompromised host   75
Laboratory diagnosis and investigations   76
   Specific diagnosis   76
   General investigations   77
Therapeutic approach to pneumonia   77
   Choice of antibiotic(s)   77
   Predisposing host abnormalities   78
   Supportive measures   78
   Specific antibiotic treatment in pneumonia   80

**Recurrent infections of the lower
respiratory tract   81**
Cystic fibrosis   81
   Antibiotic therapy   81
Bronchiectasis   82
Chronic bronchitis   82

# 4

# Respiratory infections

## INTRODUCTION

Infection of the respiratory tract is a very frequent condition and its clinical spectrum is wide-ranging from the mild nuisance caused by viral rhinitis or tracheobronchitis to the potentially serious and life-threatening pneumonia. The morbidity and economic effects resulting from respiratory infections are important. Although infections of the respiratory tract can afflict everyone, those with chronic bronchitis from smoking and with deficiencies in lung–host defences and immunity are more prone. In addition, an increasing number of respiratory infections is now occurring within the hospital environment, particularly within the intensive care unit, often with organisms resistant to commonly-used antibiotics. Lower respiratory tract infections, in particular pneumonias, continue to be an important cause of death.

In this chapter, emphasis will be placed on bacterial infections and on the use of antibiotics in their treatment. Tuberculosis and infections presenting in patients with acquired immunodeficiency syndrome (AIDS) will be discussed separately in the next chapter because of their increasing prevalence.

## ANTIBIOTICS USED IN RESPIRATORY INFECTIONS

The number of antibiotics available to treat respiratory infections has increased dramatically over the past 10 years and this has partly stood up to the challenge of new bacterial infections particularly occurring in immunocompromised patients and of emerging organisms resistant to already-established antibiotics such as penicillins. Treatment is very often initiated before results of bacterial culture are available and therefore therapeutic regimes are usually empirical for many patients with serious respiratory infections. A thorough knowledge of the more established antibiotics and of the new generations of antibiotics is necessary to the practising physician confronted with respiratory infections, particularly of the lower respiratory tract. The antibiotics used to treat respiratory infections may be classified according to their mechanism of action (Box 4.1).

## Penicillins

The penicillins which inhibit bacterial cell-wall synthesis are one of the most important group of antibiotics and new derivatives of the basic penicillin nucleus continue to be produced. The penicillins can be classified according to their spectrum of antimicrobial activities.

1. Penicillin G and Penicillin V are highly active against gram-positive cocci. Because they are hydrolysed by $\beta$-lactamases which are enzymes capable of hydrolysing penicillins, they are inactive against *Staphylococcus aureus*, a producer of the $\beta$-lactamase.

2. Penicillinase-resistant penicillins include methicillin and cloxacillin and are active against penicillinase-producing *Staphylococcus aureus*.

3. Ampicillin and amoxycillin have a broader spectrum of activity than Penicillin G and are active against gram-negative bacteria such as *Haemophilus influenzae*, *Escherichia coli* and *Proteus mirabilis*.

4. Carbenicillin, ticarcillin and azlocillin, in addition to being active against these gram-negative bacteria, also have activity against *Pseudomonas*, *Enterobacter* and *Proteus* species. Piperacillin also has activity against *Klebsiella* and certain other gram-negative bacteria.

The penicillins in the last two categories are readily hydrolysed by broad-spectrum $\beta$-lactamases that are frequently produced by many gram-negative bacteria. Clavulanic acid is an antibiotic that has little useful activity but is a potent inhibitor of many $\beta$-lactamase enzymes. It is available in combination with anoxycillin or ticarcillin. The combination of amoxycillin and clavulanic acid is active against $\beta$-lactamase producing bacteria that are resistant to amoxycillin such as *Staphylococcus aureus*, some strains of *Escherichia coli* and *Haemophilus influenzae*.

In general, penicillins achieve therapeutic concentrations readily in tissues and in secretions such as pleural fluid. The penicillins have minimal direct toxicity. By far the most com-

---

**Box 4.1    Classification of antibiotics by mechanism of action**

| Mechanism of action | Antibiotics | Mechanism of action | Antibiotics |
|---|---|---|---|
| Inhibition of synthesis or damage to cell wall | Penicillins Cephalosporins Monobactams Carbapenems Vancomycin | Inhibition of synthesis or metabolism of nucleic acids | Quinolones Rifampicin |
| | | Inhibition of protein synthesis | Aminoglycosides Tetracycline Chloramphenicol Erythromycin Clindamycin Fusidic acid |
| Inhibition of synthesis or damage damage to cytoplasmic membrane | Polymyxin | | |
| | | Interference with folic acid metabolism | Sulphonamides Trimethoprim |

mon adverse effects are hypersensitivity reactions including maculopapular rash, urticaria, fever, serum sickness and anaphylaxis.

## Cephalosporins

The cephalosporins have a similar mechanism of antibacterial action as the penicillins, and have been arbitrarily classified by 'generations', based on general features of antimicrobial activity. The first generation cephalosporins such as cephalexin and ceftazidine show good activity against gram-positive bacteria but lesser activity against gram-negative bacteria. The second generation cephalosporins such as *cefoxitine, cefuroxime* and *cephamandole* have some increased activity against gram-negative bacteria such as *Escherichia coli*, *Klebsiella pneumonia* and *Proteus mirabilis*. Cefoxitine has reliable activity against anaerobes. The third generation cephalosporins such as ceftazidime, cefsulodin, and cefotaxime are mainly characterised by their increased resistance to β-lactamases and by their broad range of activity against the gram-negative bacteria and limited activity against gram-positive bacteria. *Pseudomonas aeruginosa* is highly susceptible to ceftazidime and cefsulodin. Cefotaxine and ceftazidime have proved particularly useful in treating hospital-acquired pneumonias particularly when broad-spectrum cover is required.

Cephalosporins are particularly useful as alternatives to penicillins for many infections in patients who cannot tolerate penicillins. However, they share with the penicillins a similar propensity to hypersensitivity reactions which is related to the sharing of the β-lactam structure. They are potentially nephrotoxic but to a lesser degree than the aminoglycosides and at the recommended doses, nephrotoxicity is rare.

## Aminoglycosides

The aminoglycoside antibiotics such as gentamycin, tobramycin, and amikacin, are used primarily to treat infections caused by aerobic gram-negative bacteria by interfering with protein synthesis. They have limited activity against gram-positive bacteria. They are used in combination with a broader spectrum penicillin or cephalosporin to treat suspected gram-negative respiratory infections, in particular pneumonias, especially those due to *Pseudomonas aeruginosa*, *Enterobacter*, *Klebsiella* and *Serratia*. However, gentamycin- and tobramycin-resistant strains of these gram-negative bacteria have emerged in hospitals. This resistance arises from mutations affecting proteins in the bacterial ribosome, the target for aminoglycoside action.

The aminoglycosides are not absorbed from the gut and must be given by injection. Excretion is mainly via the kidneys and accumulation occurs in renal impairment; dosage adjustment according to blood levels is mandatory. The important side-effects are ototoxicity and nephrotoxicity which occur most commonly in the elderly and in patients with renal failure. Aminoglycosides may impair neuromuscular transmission and should not be given to patients with myasthenia gravis.

## Macrolides

Erythromycin, clarithromycin and azithromycin are macrolides which inhibit protein synthesis in bacteria and have a similar spectrum of activity to that of penicillin. They are useful as alternatives in penicillin-allergic patients but are also active against *Mycoplasma pneumonia*, *Legionella pneumophila* and *Chlamydia pneumona*.

Erythromycin is adequately absorbed from the upper intestinal tract and inactivated by gastric acid. Clarithromycin is approximately 100 times more acid stable and consequently has a higher bioavailability than erythromycin. Erythromycin is concentrated in the liver and excreted in the bile. Nausea, vomiting and diarrhoea are relatively common side-effects, requiring discontinuation in 10–20% of patients. Cholestatic hepatitis is another striking side-effect also presenting with nausea, vomiting and abdominal pain. Allergic reactions such as fever, eosinophilia and skin rashes may also occur.

## Trimethoprim-sulphamethoxazole (Co-trimoxazole)

The antimicrobial activity of the combination of trimethoprim, a diaminopyrimidine, and sulphamethoxazole, a sulphonamide, results from its actions at two different steps of the pathway for the synthesis of folic acid. The antibacterial spectrum of trimethoprim is similar to that of sulphamethoxazole with activity against most gram-negative and gram-positive bacteria. Resistance may develop when it is used alone. *Pseudomonas aeruginosa*, *Bacteroides fragilis* and enterococci are usually resistant to trimethoprim alone. However, there is a synergistic interaction between trimethoprim and sulphamethoxazole even for certain bacteria which are resistant to both such as penicillinase-producing *Staphylococcus aureus*. Thus, a whole range of gram-negative bacteria such as *Enterobacter*, *Proteus* species, *Escherichia coli* is sensitive to co-trimoxazole. *Streptococcus pneumonia* and many strains of *Staphylococcus aureus* are also inhibited. Co-trimoxazole is probably best used for treating acute exacerbations of chronic bronchitis due to *Haemophilus influenzae* and *Streptococcus pneumonia*. Trimethoprim can be used alone. Co-trimoxazole is also effective for pneumonias caused by *Pneumocystis carinii* (Ch. 5). Co-trimoxazole should be avoided in the treatment of streptococcal pharyngitis because it does not eradicate the infection. Acute otitis media in children and acute maxillary sinusitis in adults caused by *Haemophilus influenzae* or *Streptococcus pneumonia* respond well to co-trimoxazole.

The pharmacokinetic profiles of sulphamethoxazole and trimethoprim are matched in order to achieve a constant ratio of 20 to 1 in blood and tissues. Side-effects of co-trimoxazole include those seen with sulphonamides such as erythema multiforme (Stevens–Johnson syndrome), renal failure and bone marrow depression. Co-trimoxazole may induce folate deficiency in the elderly and the chronic sick patient and it is probably best to use an alternative antibiotic in the elderly. It should be avoided in pregnancy.

## Tetracyclines

Tetracyclines are bacteriostatic antibiotics which inhibit bacterial protein synthesis. They possess a wide range of antimicrobial activity against gram-positive and gram-negative bacteria, and are also effective against rickettsiae, mycoplasma and chlamydiae. The tetracyclines in common use are oxytetracycline, chlortetracycline, demeclocycline and doxycycline. They are used for acute exacerbations of chronic bronchitis because of their activity against *Haemophilus influenzae*, and for the treatment *Mycoplasma pneumoniae* and psittacosis.

Tetracyclines may cause gastrointestinal upsets and phototoxicity. They stain developing teeth and are incorporated into growing bone. Thus, they should be avoided in children and during pregnancy. The excretion of tetracyclines is significantly affected in renal impairment, with the exception of doxycycline which is mostly excreted in faeces. They are therefore contraindicated in renal failure with the exception of doxycycline.

## Quinolones

Fluorinated 4-quinolones such as norfloxacin, ofloxacin and ciprofloxacin are relatively new antibiotics with broad antimicrobial activity against *Staphylococcus aureus*, *Haemophilus influenzae*, *Branhamella catarrhalis* and *Pseudomonas aeruginosa*. They show less activity against streptococci and anaerobic bacteria. Quinolones inhibit the bacterial enzyme DNA gyrase, which is responsible for the continuous introduction of negative supercoils into DNA, and thus prevent bacteria from accommodating their long chromosomes within the cell envelope. Because of this novel action, quinolones do not appear to be susceptible to resistance mechanisms associated with the transfer of plasmids, but emergence of resistant strains (e.g. to *Pseudomonas aeruginosa*) has already been reported. These quinolones, particularly ciprofloxacin, should be reserved for the treatment of respiratory infections caused by organisms resistant to standard drugs. For example, ciprofloxacin could be used in exacerbations of chronic bronchitis with gram-negative bacteria such as *Haemophilus influenzae* and *Branhamella catarrhalis* where ampicillin, amoxycillin or erythromycin has already been unsuccessful. Ciprofloxacin therapy can be effective in chest infections due to *Pseudomous aeruginosa* in patients with cystic fibrosis when administered orally.

Ciprofloxacin is well absorbed after oral administration. It penetrates human tissues well, with high levels achieved in pulmonary, bronchial and bone tissues, and also in phagocytic cells. Antacids reduce its bioavailability considerably. About half of the drug is excreted unchanged in the urine. Quinolones can produce nausea, abdominal pain and headaches. They are not recommended for children or pregnant women because of the possibility of damage to cartilage. Dosage of theophylline should be reduced or stopped while on quinolones.

## New β-lactams

Aztreonam, a monobactam (a single-ringed β-lactam), comes from a new class of antibiotic with high activity limited to gram-negative enteric bacilli such as enterobacteria and *Pseudomonas aeruginosa* with no activity against gram-positive and anaerobic bacteria. Side-effects are similar to those of other β-lactams with less potential for developing hypersensitivity. Aztreonam is excreted unchanged in the urine.

Imipenem, the first of a new β-lactam class, the carbapenems, has a broader range of activity than the cephalosporins against anaerobic and gram-positive bacteria, including *Bacteroides*. It is stable to β-lactamase. It is partly inactivated in the kidney and is administered with cilastatin which is a specific enzyme inhibitor of its renal metabolism.

## Vancomycin

Vancomycin is a tricyclic glycopeptide with primary activity against gram-positive bacteria. It should be reserved for treating pneumonia or empyema due to penicillin-resistant *Staphylococcus aureus*. Vancomycin is administered intravenously. Untoward reactions include hypersensitivity reactions, ototoxicity and nephrotoxicity. Caution needs to be exercised in patients with renal impairment and when administered concomitantly with aminoglycosides.

## Clindamycin

Clindamycin has a profile of activity against gram-positive cocci including penicillin-resistant staphylococci and also against many anaerobes, particularly *Bacteroides fragilis*. Clindamycin concentrates well in bone and is excreted in the urine and bile. Clindamycin is an alternative to penicillin for the treatment of aspiration pneumonia or bacterial abscesses due to anaerobes, particularly *Bacteroides fragilis*. The most serious toxic effect of clindamycin is pseudomembranous colitis, which may be fatal.

## UPPER RESPIRATORY TRACT INFECTIONS

Upper respiratory tract infections represent one of the most common categories of infectious diseases, usually manifested by influenza-like illnesses and common colds. Probably between 10 to 20% of all general practice consultations relate to infections of the upper respiratory tract. Infectious agents may cause disease in the nose, paranasal sinuses, the middle ear, and the pharynx. Although viruses are the most common agents to infect these structures, bacterial pathogens are often involved (Table 4.1) and appropriate antibiotics must be given.

**Table 4.1   Bacterial pathogens in upper respiratory tract infection**

| Organism | Acute rhinitis and sinusitis | Acute otitis media |
|---|---|---|
| Haemophilus influenzae | Common (30%) | Common (30%) |
| Streptococcus pneumoniae | Common (40%) | Common (35%) |
| Streptococcus pyogenes | Less common (5–10%) | Less common (2%) |
| Branhamella catarrhalis | Less common (5%) | Less common (3%) |
| Staphylococcus aureus | Uncommon (2%) | Less common (5%) |
| Anaerobes | Uncommon (1%) | Less common (7%) |

# Rhinitis

By far the vast majority of acute rhinitis is due to viruses with rhinoviruses accounting for up to 30% of cases, and with the involvement of other viruses such as parainfluenzae, influenza, respiratory syncytial virus and adenoviruses. Acute rhinitis may also be caused by bacteria such as *Mycoplasma pneumoniae* and the recently-described *Chlamydia pneumoniae*. The symptoms of acute rhinitis or of the common cold include nasal congestion, sneezing, nasal discharge, sore throat and reproductive cough. This is generally a self-limiting illness and treatment is directed towards the relief of symptoms.

# Sinusitis

The most common cause of acute bacterial sinusitis include *Streptoccocus pneumoniae*, *Haemophilus influenzae* and oral anaerobes. *Staphylococcus aureus* and *Branhamella catarrhalis* may also be involved and these may produce β-lactamase. Predisposing factors for the development of acute sinusitis include a recent viral infection of the upper respiratory tract, allergic rhinitis, trauma to the orofacial area and recent dental procedure involving the maxillae. The presenting features are usually facial pain and purulent discharge, sometimes associated with nasal congestion and pain on mastication. There may be a low-grade fever. Involvement of the maxillary and frontal sinuses usually produce localised pain aggravated by movement or by percussion. Ethmoid or sphenoid sinusitis may produce retro-orbital pain, sometimes severe at night. Complications of acute sinusitis can be serious, depending on the site of the sinusitis. Extension of the infection from frontal and ethmoid sinuses can lead to a subdural or intracranial abscess. Cavernous sinus thrombosis is a life-threatening emergency.

Antibiotic treatment of acute sinusitis is justified, and initial therapy should include amoxycillin or co-trimoxazole. The tetracycline, vibramycin, achieves high concentrations in the sinuses and is also an acceptable choice. If resistance to ampicillin is encountered, a new β-lactamase resistant antibiotic such as co-amoxiclav (amoxycillin with clavulanic acid) or a second-generation cephalosporin such as cefuroxime should be used.

## Pharyngitis

Sore throat is a common complaint and the majority of cases of acute pharyngitis is accounted for by respiratory viruses. Bacterial causes of acute pharyngitis include group A β-haemolytic streptococcus, Haemophilus influenzae, Corynebacterium diphtheriae and Fusobacterium. A sudden onset of high fever and severe throat pain associated with patchy exudates on the tonsils and posterior pharynx are typical of a β-haemolytic streptococcal infection. Corynebacterium diphtheriae infection is unusual in the UK and is characterised by the presence of a membrane on the tonsils, extending to the uvula and soft palate, sometimes associated with fever, hoarseness, shortness of breath and tachycardia in more severe cases. Both Corynebacterium diphtheriae and β-haemolytic streptococcus should be treated with parenteral penicillin or erythromycin, with the administration of diphtheria antitoxin for diphtherial pharyngitis after a cutaneous test dose.

Mucosal ulcerations in the pharynx in association with sore throat may be seen with Herpes simplex virus, Coxsackie A, and fusobacterial infections. Cytomegalovirus and Toxoplasma gondii can both give rise to a sore throat, fever, lymphadenopathy and lymphocytosis.

## Laryngotracheitis and epiglottitis

Laryngotracheitis in adults is usually secondary to viruses and presents with hoarseness, a persistent dry cough and upper respiratory symptoms. In children, stridor may be a presenting feature of laryngotracheitis which is usually due to parainfluenza virus. However, bacterial tracheitis with Staphylococcus aureus or Haemophilus influenzae may also produce fever and stridor. Progressive upper respiratory compromise must be promptly treated with the aim of reducing airway oedema, using inhaled adrenergic agents and systemic corticosteroids.

Acute epiglottitis is a medical emergency, usually presenting in a similar way to laryngotracheitis. Haemophilus influenzae is the usual infective bacterial agent. Amoxycillin preferably with clavulanic acid is the antibiotic of choice. A β-lactamase resistant cephalosporin or co-trimoxazole may be used as alternatives.

## Otitis media

Acute bacterial otitis media usually presents with severe ear pain associated with fever, tenderness over the mastoid and hearing impairment. The tympanic membrane appears red and bulging, and may sometimes perforate. The most common bacteria isolated are Streptococcus pneumoniae, Haemophilus influenzae and Brahamella catarrhalis, but viruses such as respiratory syncytial virus have been obtained. The antibiotics often used are either amoxycillin, ampicillin or co-trimoxazole.

## LOWER RESPIRATORY TRACT INFECTIONS

### Pneumonias

Despite the advent of antibiotics and improved methods for diagnosis, pneumonia continues to be a significant medical problem and to contribute to a large number of deaths. In the UK, deaths from pneumonia are approximately 10 times more frequent than those caused by all other infections added together. In the USA, pneumonia is the third most common hospital-acquired infection, after urinary tract and wound infections. This continuing problem of pneumonia may relate to the change in the patient population at risk such as the increasing number of aged and debilitated, and of immunosuppressed patients, and to the involvement of a different spectrum of infective organisms. These 'new' types of pneumonias present a continuing challenge to the clinician concerning diagnosis and treatment, together with the frequent emergence of antimicrobial resistance of well-known bacteria.

---

**Box 4.2  Bacterial causes of pneumonia**

**Community acquired:**

*Streptococcus pneumoniae*
*Mycoplasma pneumoniae*
*Haemophilus influenzae*
*Legionella species*
*Chlamydia psittaci (less common)*
*Staphylococcus aureus*

**Hospital acquired:**

*Staphylococcus aureus*
*Pseudomonas aeruginosa*
*Enteric gram-negative bacilli*

**Aspiration:**

*Fusobacterium species*
*Bacteroides melaninogenicus*
*Peptostreptococci*

**Immunosuppressed:**

*Pneumocystis carinii*
*Legionella pneumophila*
*Cryptococcus*
*Nocardia*

---

## Clinical approach to pneumonia

Pneumonia must be distinguished clinically from acute bronchitis which usually presents with cough and sputum production in the absence of a fever and in association with upper respiratory tract symptoms. Acute bronchitis is usually secondary to infection with viruses associated with upper respiratory tract infections. Patients with pneumonia usually present with symptoms of fever and productive cough, sometimes associated with pleuritic pain, and with evidence of consolidation on chest examination. The chest radiograph is useful in confirming the diagnosis and documenting the extent of the pneumonia, and the presence of complications such as a pleural effusion or of cavitation. Distinction between a bacterial and a viral pneumonia may be difficult, although the mucoid character of sputum in a viral pneumonia may be different from the more purulent nature of a bacterial pneumonia. This may particularly arise in patients with chronic lung disease.

In the patient with a likely diagnosis of pneumonia, it is important to determine rapidly the incriminating pathogen from all the information available so that subsequent treatment and outcome is optimised by administration of the proper antibiotic(s). Patients who die of pneumonia have most often not received appropriate antibiotics when first seen. The organisms responsible for pneumonias may differ depending upon the circumstances under which the patient presents (Box 4.2).

### Community-acquired pneumonia

Community-acquired pneumonia is most commonly caused by *Streptococcus pneumoniae*, but other less common bacterial causes include *Haemophilus influenzae*, *Legionella* species and *Staphylococcus aureus*. Up to 15–20% of causes are due to atypical pneumonia particularly *Mycoplasma pneumoniae* which occurs commonly in young adults. Legionnaire's disease occurs spasmodically and in outbreaks throughout the year but is more common in late summer and early autumn. Gram-negative bacterial infections are unusual in the community setting.

Predisposing factors to pneumonia acquired in the community can often be identified. Old age, recent viral infection, diabetes mellitus, chronic renal failure and malignancy form a particularly high-risk group. A history of contact with birds may lead to the suspicion of psittacosis (due to *Chlamydia psittaci*) or of Q fever (due to *Cloxiella burnetti*).

An abrupt onset of fever, shaking chills with a cough productive of purulent sputum and sometimes with a pleuritic chest pain are common presenting symptoms of typical pneumonias. An additional history of recent upper respiratory tract infection may indicate bacterial superinfection, usually with *Staphylococcus aureus*. A more insidious onset with headache, sore throat, myalgias and fatigue with a persistent dry cough would normally indicate atypical pneumonia, often due to *Mycoplasma pneumoniae*, respiratory viruses and *Legionella* species.

## Hospital-acquired pneumonia

The bacterial organisms most frequently associated with hospital-acquired pneumonia are the gram-negative bacteria such as *Escherichia coli*, *Klebsiella pneumoniae*, *Pseudomonas aeruginosa* and Enterobacter species, which are often resistant to many antibiotics. The pattern of antibiotic resistance is usually specific for each hospital. *Staphylococcus aureus* is also responsible for a smaller proportion of cases. The most important predisposing factors to hospital-acquired pneumonia include endotracheal intubation or tracheostomy, which presumably cause injury to the respiratory mucosa, which is subsequently predisposed to infection. Previous prophylactic antibiotic use in hospital may also select out the growth of more resistant bacterial pathogens, especially in patients recovering from surgery.

In ill patients with hospital-acquired pneumonia, it is often difficult to establish the diagnosis clearly when specific respiratory symptoms and signs may be absent. Abnormal appearances of pulmonary infiltrates on the chest radiograph may be due to other causes from pneumonia, such as pulmonary infection, lung collapse or adult respiratory distress syndrome.

## Aspiration pneumonia

Aspiration pneumonia is usually associated with an episode of altered consciousness such as during seizures, general anaesthesia or cerebrovascular accidents or with abnormalities of oesophageal function such as dysphagia and oesophageal reflux. Aspiration pneumonia acquired within the community is usually secondary to anaerobes from the gingival crevices such as: *Bacteroides melaninogenicus*, *Fusobacterium* species and peptostreptococci. However, in the hospital setting, gram-negative bacteria and *Staphylococcus aureus* which commonly colonise the upper respiratory tract of hospitalised patients may also be involved in aspiration pneumonia.

The most common site of aspiration pneumonia is the posterior segment of the right upper lobe, with the same segment on the left less commonly affected. The apical segments of both lower lobes are next in frequency of involvement. The inhaled material is distributed according to gravity and the posture of the subject. If gastric contents are aspirated, gastric acid and enzymes are usually the primary damaging agents, followed by bacterial invasion. The initial clinical picture of aspiration pneumonia has no distinctive features apart from predisposition to aspiration and involvement of dependent segments of the lung. In many patients, tissue necrosis may lead to abscess formation or empyema after 1 or 2 weeks. Foul-smelling sputum may then be coughed up.

## Immunocompromised host

Pneumonia in the immunocompromised host is now becoming an increasingly important problem due to the effects of immunosuppressive and cytotoxic therapy in patients with solid tumours and myeloproliferative disorders, and in transplant recipients, and, more recently, in patients with the acquired immunodeficiency syndrome (AIDS) (Ch. 5). In such patients, infection of the lower respiratory tract is a common cause of morbidity and mortality, but other non-infectious pulmonary complications are also common including adverse reactions to drugs, pulmonary emboli or progression of the underlying disease.

Fever is by far the most common sign of infection and often the only sign, with absence of cough, sputum and leukocytosis. The chest radiograph may show the presence of new infiltrates. Such patients must be investigated with sputum and blood cultures, and sometimes with invasive procedures to obtain a correct diagnosis, before the institution of empiric antimicrobial therapy.

Pneumonia in the immunocompromised host may be caused by bacteria and mycobacteria, viruses, fungal and parasitic agents (Box 4.3). In patients with granulocytopenia resulting from treatment of leukaemia and lymphoproliferative disorders, infections with gram-negative bacilli (e.g. *Escherichia coli*, *Klebsiella*, *Pseudomonas aeruginosa*) as well as *Staphylococcus aureus* continue to predominate. Fungi (e.g. *Aspergillus* species, *Candida* and *Cryptococcus neoformans*) are also important pathogens particularly during treatment with broad-spectrum antibiotics. In transplant recipients, organisms which may be responsible for causing pulmonary infiltrates include cytomegalovirus, *Pneumocystis carinii*, fungi and conventional bacterial pathogens. Hospital-acquired infections with *Legionella pneumophila*, *Aspergillus* species and *Pseudomonas aeruginosa* are well documented. Infections in patients with the acquired immune deficiency syndrome (AIDS) is discussed in a separate chapter.

## Laboratory diagnosis and investigations

### Specific diagnosis

Whenever the diagnosis of pneumonia is considered, all specimens for microbiological culture should be obtained including sputum and blood cultures. Gram-staining of sputum may show predominance of a pathogenic organism such *Pneumococcus* or *Haemophilus*, and cultures of sputum specimens may yield an organism, although this is significantly reduced if the patient is already on antibiotics. More often, oropharyngeal contamination of sputum may make interpretation of sputum culture difficult. Pleural fluid if present should be sampled for bacteriological analysis.

---

**Box 4.3   Causes of pulmonary infiltrates in immunocompromised patients**

**Infectious**

*Bacterial*

Staphylococcus aureus
Drug-induced lung damage
Gram-negative bacilli
*Legionella*
*Nocardi*

*Mycobacterial*

Mycobacterium tuberculosis
Atypical mycobacteria
e.g. avium, etc

*Viral*

Cytomegalorins
Herpes simplex
Adenovirus
Varicella-zoster

*Fungal*

Cryptococcus
Aspergillus
Mucormycosis
Candida

*Parasitic*

*Pneumocystis carinii*
*Toxoplasma gondii*

**Non-infectious**

Pulmonary oedema
Radiation pneumonitis
Pulmonary haemorrhage
Pulmonary embolism
and infarction
Spread of neoplastic
condition
Kaposi's sarcoma

More invasive methods for diagnosing lower respiratory tract infection include transtracheal aspiration, fibreoptic bronchoscopy with aspiration and transbronchial or open-lung biopsy, and should be considered if the potential benefit of an accurate bacteriologic diagnosis outweighs the risks of these methods and if an urgent aetiological diagnosis is necessary.

Serological evaluation should also be considered, particularly when the bacterial agent is not readily isolated and cultured. The diagnosis of *Mycoplasma pneumoniae* infection will be supported by the presence of cold agglutinins and by complement fixation test. Serological tests are also available for diagnosing *Legionella* species, brucellosis and psittacosis, but such diagnoses are usually made retrospectively. Counterimmunoelectrophoresis of blood, sputum or urine may identify the pneumococcal antigen.

### General investigations

A *white cell count* may be markedly elevated with pyogenic pneumonia, while a near normal count is usually compatible with atypical and viral pneumonia. The *chest radiograph* should be used to document the presence and the extent of the pneumonia, although in patients with significant neutropenia the presence of pulmonary consolidation or infiltrates may be minimal. The location of pulmonary consolidation such as the posterior segment of the upper lobes or the superior segments of the lower lobe may favour

aspiration pneumonia. The presence of cavitation, pleural effusion, lymphadenopathy, and collapse may help to narrow the diagnosis. *Biochemical tests* such as abnormal liver function tests and hypoalbuminaemia may indicate the severity of the infection, as arterial blood gas estimations.

## Therapeutic approach to pneumonia

This should include: a) choice of antimicrobial agent or agents to use; b) attempt at correcting predisposing or remediable host factors and c) general supportive measures.  Patients with pneumonia should in general be treated in hospital but some with mild symptoms can be managed at home but should be admitted to hospital if there is clinical deterioration. Indications for treating pneumonia in the intensive care setting are given in Box 4.4.

### Choice of antibiotic(s)

The choice of antibiotic(s) to be used depends on the bacteria suspected and this decision will rest upon the clinical setting and the results of preliminary diagnostic tests that have been performed. Treatment must be started before laboratory confirmation of the underlying organism is obtained and in some patients, it is possible to guess the infecting bacteria with a high degree of certainty. The use of specific antibiotics to cover specific infective organisms is dealt with later. In many cases, particularly in severely ill patients and in immunocompromised patients, management should cover all bacterial pathogens appropriate to the clinical setting, and broad-spectrum coverage is indicated. Antibiotic therapy may be altered appropriately when specific pathogens have been isolated or if the condition of the patient is deteriorating without any pathogen being identified. When the aetiological agent of pneumonia has been identified, the initial regime may be changed to a drug specific for that agent. The initial choice of antibiotics for pneumonia acquired in differ-

---

**Box 4.4   Indications for intensive care of pneumonia**

Severe pneumonia with
- Arterial $pO_2$ < 8kPa despite inspired oxygen > 60%
- Arterial $pCO_2$ > 6.4 kPa
- Exhaustion, drowsiness or impaired consciousness
- Respiratory or cardiac arrest
- Shock

ent clinical settings is given below. Response to therapy should be reviewed on a regular frequent basis depending on the clinical condition and in the face of an unsatisfactory therapeutic response (Box 4.5).

## Predisposing host abnormalities

Host abnormalities in patients with pneumonia may impede recovery or predispose to further episodes of infection. Purulent collections in the pleural space or pericardium should be drained. Lung abscesses usually communicate through the upper airways and may be drained by postural drainage and by fibreoptic bronchoscopy. In some cases, for example, bronchial obstruction by a tumour must be tackled to allow drainage of any lung abscess. The possibility of oesophageal disease should be considered in patients with aspiration pneumonia, and dental problems should be appropriately treated. Advice about stopping alcohol intake should also be given.

Patients on immunosuppressive treatment and with congenital and acquired immunodefi-

ciencies are prone to lower respiratory tract infections. Stopping immunosuppressive therapy may lead to an improvement in the host defence to infections, but during periods of immunosuppression, granulocyte infusions may be used and more recently, the use of granulocyte colony stimulating factor has been tried during chemotherapy to accelerate bone marrow recovery. Immunoglobulin infusions may be used in patients with acquired immunodeficiency. Patients who have undergone splenectomy or without a functional spleen such as in sickle-cell disease are prone to fulminant pneumococcal pneumonia, and vaccination with the pneumococcal vaccine is advisable. Prophylactic antibiotic therapy can also be recommended in susceptible groups prone to lower respiratory tract infections from either immunodeficiencies or local airway disease.

## Supportive measures

General supportive measures are essential during the period when antibiotics are administered to treat the infection. Dehydration is a common feature as a result of poor oral intake and increased fluid losses associated with high fever. Electrolyte disturbance may also occur following dehydration and also may be a feature of particular pneumonias such as *Legionella pneumophila*. These defects may require intravenous therapy if patients cannot drink enough to maintain adequate hydration. Adequate calorie and nutritional intake may be necessary in patients with complications from pneumonia such as empyema or abscess formation.

Supplemental oxygen is necessary in patients with documented hypoxaemia, and for those with persistent hypoxaemia despite supplemental oxygen (arterial oxygen less than 8 kPa) or for those who are exhausted, intubation and mechanical ventilation will be required. Renal failure may be a complication of pneumonia and should be managed energetically as appropriate.

Physiotherapy is useful with pneumonia which occurs in patients with chronic bronchitis

---

**Box 4.5   Causes of unsatisfactory response of pneumonia**

1.  Diagnosis incorrect: reconsider

e.g. pulmonary oedema
   pulmonary eosinophilia
   Wegener's granulomatosis
   organising pneumonia

2.  Organism resistant to antibiotics

e.g. ampicillin-resistant *Haemophilus influenzae* or
   *Staphylococcus aureus*
   undiagnosed immunodeficiency with
   *Pneumocystis carinii*
   undiagnosed pulmonary tuberculosis

3.  Development of complications

e.g. lung abscess (anaerobic infection)
   empyema
   pulmonary embolism
   side-effects of antibiotics (e.g. drug fever)

**Table 4.2  Antibiotics for specific bacteria causing pneumonia**

| Organism | Antibiotics | Dose and frequency | |
|---|---|---|---|
| Streptococcus pneumoniae | Penicillin G | 0.6–1.2 g | 6 hourly i.v. |
| | Amoxycillin | 500 mg | 8 hourly oral or i.v. |
| | Erythromycin | 500–1000 mg | 6 hourly i.v. |
| | | or 250–500 mg | 6 hourly oral |
| | Cefuroxime | 1.5 g | 8 hourly i.v. |
| | or | | |
| | Cefotamine | 2 g | 8 hourly i.v. |
| Staphylococcus aureus | Flucloxacillin | 2 g | 6 hourly i.v. |
| | ±Fusidic acid | 500–1000 mg | 8 hourly i.v. |
| | Vancomycin | 500 mg | 6 hourly i.v. |
| | | or 1000 mg | 12 hourly i.v. |
| Haemophilus influenzae | Ampicillin | 500 mg | 6 hourly oral or i.v. |
| | Amoxycillin | 500 mg | 8 hourly oral or i.v. |
| | (or Amoxycillin with clavulanic acid) | | |
| | Co-trimoxazole | 960 mg | 12 hourly oral or i.v. |
| | Cefuroxime | 1.5 g | 8 hourly i.v. |
| Legionella | Erythromycin | 500–1000 mg | 6 hourly i.v. or oral |
| | ±Rifampicin | 600 mg | 12 hourly i.v. |
| | or | | |
| | ±Ciprofloxacin | 200 mg | 8 hourly i.v. |
| Mycoplasma pneumoniae | Erythromycin | 500–1000 mg | 6 hourly i.v.or oral |
| Chlamydia psittaci | Tetracycline | | |
| Q fever | | 250–500 mg | 6 hourly i.v. or oral |
| Anaerobes | Penicillin G | 0.6–1.2 g | 6 hourly i.v. |
| | or | | |
| | Amoxycillin | 500 mg | 8 hourly i.v. |
| | plus | | |
| | Metronidazole | 500 mg | 8 hourly oral |
| | | | 8 hourly i.v. or oral |
| | or | | |
| | Clindamycin | up to 450 mg | 6 hourly i.v. or oral |
| Pseudomonas aeruginosa | Gentamicin | 80–120 mg | 8 hourly i.v. |
| | or | | |
| | Tobramycin | 3.5 mg/kg | in divided doses every 6-8 hours |
| | or | | |
| | Amikacin | 1.5 mg/kg | in divided doses every 12 hours |
| Klebsiella pneumoniae | Ticarcillin | 15–20 g | daily in 6-hourly doses |
| | or | | |
| | Azlocillin | 2.5 g | every 8 hours |
| | or | | |
| | Cefotaxime | 1 g | 12 hourly i.v. |
| | or | | |
| | Ceftazidine | 1–2 g | 8 hourly i.v. |
| | or | | |
| | Carbenicillin | 5 g | 6 hourly i.m. or i.v. |

or bronchiectasis, or with lung abscess. Otherwise, physiotherapy may cause fatigue to an already sick patient. Bronchodilators are indicated if there is evidence of bronchospasm.

### Specific antibiotic treatment in pneumonia

A summary of the antibiotics usually recommended for specific bacterial organisms causing pneumonia is given in Table 4.2.

*Community-acquired.* The sudden onset of lobar consolidation in the community associated with a gram-stain of expectorated sputum of gram-positive elongated diplococci would suggest that penicillin treatment is appropriate. However, in a patient with long-standing chronic bronchitis such a presentation in the community may be secondary to *Haemophilus influenzae*, particularly if the gram-stain shows gram-negative bacilli, when ampicillin or co-trimoxazole may be more appropriate. In practice, ampicillin or one of its derivatives is a good choice. When an atypical pneumonia such as with *Mycoplasma pneumonia* or *Legionella pneumophilia* is suspected, erythromycin should be considered. In the patient with severe community-acquired pneumonia of indeterminate cause, the best combination for good initial cover would be intravenous amoxycillin, plus erythromycin. In milder cases, oral therapy with amoxycillin and erythromycin may be considered. If staphylococcal pneumonia is also suspected (particularly during an influenza epidemic), flucloxacillin or another anti-staphylococcal agent such as vancomycin or fusidic acid should be added. Alternatively, a second or third generation cephalosporin such as cefuroxime or cefotamine could be considered.

*Hospital-acquired.* Empiric treatment of hospital-acquired pneumonia should include combination or broad-spectrum antibiotics as initial therapy because of the variety of potential pathogens such as aerobic gram-negative bacilli (e.g. *Pseudomonas aeruginosa, Serratia marcescens,* acinetobacter) as well as *Staphylococcus aureus.* The combination antibiotic regimes generally include an aminoglycoside such as gentamicin or tobramycin with either a third-generation cephalosporin such as cefotaxime or ceftazidime for broad cover against gram-negative bacteria or a broad-spectrum penicillin such as ticarcillin or azlocillin with particular activity against *Pseudomonas.*

The use of single-agent antibiotics for hospital-acquired infections particularly with broad-spectrum $\beta$-lactam antibiotics has also been advocated but it is still best to combine these agents with an aminoglycoside because of their synergistic effects particularly against *Pseudomonas aeruginosa.*

Pneumonias due to enterobacter, *Serratia* and acinetobacter are particularly difficult to treat with the development of resistance during treatment. Enterobacter and *Serratia* infections should be treated with a third-generation cephalosporin plus an aminoglycoside in high dosage. Imipenem may also be used.

*Aspiration pneumonia.* In aspiration pneumonia, antibiotics effective against various anaerobic bacteria should be included. Penicillin G is active against a wide range of anaerobes except against the *Bacteroides fragilis* group or other $\beta$-lactamase producing anaerobes. If the patient is seriously ill, clindamycin or metronidazole may be added to Penicillin G to cover these penicillin-resistant groups. Clindamycin may induce diarrhoea and clostridium difficile colitis. Erythromycin or vancomycin may be used instead of Penicillin G in case of penicillin allergy, and these antibiotics also have the advantage of covering other bacteria such as any suspected staphylococcal infections in the case of vancomycin.

For hospital-acquired aspiration pneumonia, a combination of an aminoglycoside with clindamycin or penicillin should be used to cover in addition to anaerobes gram-negative bacilli such as *Klebsiella pneumoniae* and *Pseudomonas aeruginosa.* Treatment may be required for 3 to 6 weeks, particularly if empyema or lung abscess occurs. Bronchoscopy is useful to remove particulate matter from the respiratory tract. Whether prophylactic antibiotics are useful in acid aspiration pneumonia is not known and the value of corticosteroids is also unclear.

*Immunocompromised patients.* Because there is a whole host of infectious and of non-infectious causes of pneumonic consolidation or infiltrates in immunocompromised patients, it is difficult to summarise a single approach. If bacterial infection cannot be excluded, empiric antibiotics should be immediately started, usually to cover staphylococcus and resistant gram-negative bacilli such as those advocated for covering hospital-acquired pneumonia. Vancomycin may be added for covering staphylococcus. Suspicion of tuberculosis should prompt appropriate antituberculous therapy (Ch. 6). When *Pneumocystis carinii* is suggested by the clinical setting and by diffuse bilateral pulmonary infiltrates, appropriate therapy such as co-trimoxazole should be instituted (Ch. 6). Further antibiotic therapy may be determined by the results of specific, usually invasive tests. Thus, amphotericin B may be added for possible fungal infections and erythromycin for Legionnaire's disease.

# RECURRENT INFECTIONS OF THE LOWER RESPIRATORY TRACT

## Cystic fibrosis (CF)

One of the leading causes of morbidity and mortality in CF is due to progressive pulmonary failure caused by chronic lower respiratory tract infections starting in early childhood. Initially, infants may present with recurrent pneumonias, particularly with staphylococcal infections, and there may be persistence of fever, productive cough and chest pain. Accumulating lung damage may lead progressively to secondary pulmonary hypertension. There may be evidence of bronchial changes with goblet cell hyperplasia, acute and chronic pulmonary infiltrates, bronchiectasis and mucopurulent plugging of airways.

The initial pulmonary bacterial pathogen is usually *Staphylococcus aureus* which colonises the sputum of CF patients intermittently. *Pseudomonas aeruginosa* is sometimes isolated in the early stage of the disease and it is possible that staphylococcal-induced airway and lung disease predisposes to subsequent *Pseudomonas aeruginosa* colonisation. Extracellular alginate produced by mucoid strains of *Pseudomonas aeruginosa* enhances the colonisation of the lower respiratory tract. Patients with moderate to severe disease are commonly infected with such colonial forms. Other *Pseudomonas* species such as *Pseudomonas cepaciae* have been isolated from sputum of CF patients, but its pathological significance is not clear. *Haemophilus influenzae* is often isolated in association with *Pseudomonas aeruginosa* from sputum of CF patients with established pulmonary infection. The pathogenicity of other organisms such as *Candida albicans*, mycobacteria and *Aspergillus* species found in CF sputum is not certain.

### Antibiotic therapy

Infections with *Haemophilus influenzae* can be treated with amoxycillin, co-trimoxazole, erythromycin and chloramphenicol. Infections with *Staphylococcus aureus* should be treated with flucoxacillin, with the addition of sodium fusidate if the infection is serious. In patients who are allergic to penicillin, erythromycin is less established particularly as the respiratory tract of many adult patients with cystic fibrosis is colonised with *Pseudomonas aeruginosa*. Although it is usual practice to treat in the presence of increasing symptoms (cough, sputum or breathlessness and fever), some clinicians advocate treating every 3 months irrespective of symptoms. *Pseudomonas aeruginosa* infection should be treated with a combination of aminoglycoside (tobramycin, gentamicin or amikacin) and either a penicillin with activity against *Pseudomonas* (carbenicillin, ticarcillin oralocillin) or a third generation cephalosporin (ceftazidine or cefsulodin). Patients requiring frequent treatment with these antibiotics may need an indwelling intravenous catheter and be taught to inject themselves with these antibiotics. Each course of treatment should be for a minimum of 10–14 days. More recently ciprofloxacin, an orally active quinolone, has been shown to be effective by the intravenous route and is now widely used for the treatment of infections with *Pseudomonas aeruginosa* in CF patients. Whether this will lead to emergence of resistant organisms is not known.

The use of daily nebulised carbenicillin and gentamicin may reduce the frequency of hospital admissions in CF patients infected chronically with *Pseudomonas aeruginosa*. Colomycin has also been used. This treatment is expensive and time-consuming for the patient, and should be tried in selected CF patients who need frequent hospital admissions and show deterioration in lung function.

## Bronchiectasis

Bronchiectasis is a disease characterised by permanent dilation of the bronchi, associated with many recognised conditions such as immunoglobulin deficiencies, defects in mucociliary clearance, cystic fibrosis, childhood infections such as measles and whooping cough and allergic bronchopulmonary aspergillosis. Patients with bronchiectasis have bronchial damage, excess mucus production and impaired clearance. In most patients, the presence of bacterial infections and inflammation is intermittent. However, there is a subgroup of patients in whom bacterial colonisation, neutrophil recruitment and inflammation are continually present. These subjects persistently produce frank purulent sputum, probably due to a vicious circle enhanced by the presence of neutrophil products which cause further tissue-damage. The secretions of patients with bronchiectasis are often colonised with bacteria such as *Haemophilus influenzae* and *Streptococcus pneumoniae*. Use of broad spectrum antibiotics in addition to reducing bacterial colonisation leads to a decrease in neutrophil products such as elastase and in protein leakage into the airways.

Antibiotics have been the mainstay of treatment of infective exacerbations in bronchiectasis and consist of broad-spectrum antibiotics, usually amoxycillin or co-trimoxazole administered over 14 days. The choice of antibiotics will

finally depend on the results of sputum culture. Amoxycillin has been shown to penetrate in bronchial secretions better than ampicillin. In some patients, high doses of amoxycillin (up to 6 g per day for 10 days) may be necessary to control an infective episode. Inhaled amoxyillin may be useful in some cases. The emergence of *Pseudomonas* infection in the bronchiectatic airway should be managed in a similar fashion to that of the patient with cystic fibrosis.

Other important aspects of the treatment of bronchiectasis include daily postural drainage and bronchodilator therapy if there is evidence of reversible airways obstruction. Other conditions associated with bronchiectasis may need particular attention e.g. immunoglobulin deficiency.

## Chronic bronchitis (see Ch. 2)

Chronic bronchitis is defined as a condition in which there is coughing up of sputum for at least 3 months of the year for 2 consecutive years, for which no other cause such as bronchiectasis is evident. Hypersecretion of mucus may predispose to recurrent chest infections and progressive airflow obstruction may occur. Upper respiratory virus infections such as rhinovirus and parainfluenza virus may lead to acute exacerbations of bronchitis in such patients and may predispose them to secondary upper and lower respiratory tract bacterial infections with almost invariably *Haemophilus influenzae* or *Streptococcus pneumoniae*. More recently, *Branhamella catarrhalis* has been isolated with increasing frequency. The development of respiratory bacterial infection is usually recognised by the development of purulent sputum.

These episodes should be promptly treated with a week's course of an antibiotic, usually a tetracycline or ampicillin or amoxycillin or co-trimoxazole. Co-trimoxazole is now considered to be no more effective than trimethroprim alone. Infections caused by organisms known to be resistant to amoxycillin because of $\beta$-lactamase production may be treated with a combination of amoxycillin and clavulanic acid or a second-generation cephalosporin such as cefuroxime. Prompt treatment of such exacerbations can be achieved by asking patients with chronic bronchitis to keep a supply of antibiotics at home to be taken at the first sign of an exacerbation. Long-term chemoprophylaxis is not recommended except for some selected patients such as those experiencing recurrent exacerbations in the winter months.

## FURTHER READING

British Thoracic Society 1987 Community-acquired pneumonia in adults in British hospitals 1982–1983: a survey of aetiology, mortality, prognostic factors and outcome. Quarterly Journal of Medicine 62: 195–220

Harrison B D W, Farr B M, Connolly C K, MacFarlane B M, Selkon J B, Bartlett C L R 1987. The hospital management of community-acquired pneumonia. Journal of the Royal College of London 21: 267–296

Levison M E (ed) 1984 The pneumonias: clinical approaches to infectious diseases of the lower respiratory tract. J. Wright, Massachusetts

MacFarlane J T 1987 Treatment of lower respiratory tract infections. Lancet 2: 1446–1449

Pennington J E (ed) 1983 Respiratory infections: diagnosis and management. Raven Press, New York

CHAPTER CONTENTS

**Tests used for the diagnosis of pulmonary disease in HIV positive patients   86**
Non-invasive tests   86
Tests for aetiological diagnosis   86
    Induced sputum   87
    Bronchoscopy   87
    Open-lung biopsy   88

**Therapy of pulmonary infections in HIV positive patients   88**
    Antiretroviral treatment   88
    Other antiretroviral strategies   89

*Pneumocystis carinii*   89
    Treatment of *Pneumocystis carinii* pneumonia   89
    Causes of deterioration in patients with *Pneumocystis carinii* pneumonia   92
    General measures in AIDS patients with severe pneumonia   92
    Bacterial infections   92
    Mycobacterial infections   93
    Cytomegalovirus infection   93
    Prevention of lung infections   94

# 5

# Opportunistic infections in the acquired immune deficiency syndrome

The latest World Health Organisation figures for the number of people worldwide with the acquired immune deficiency syndrome (AIDS) suggests that more than one and a half million people have the disease. The number of people who have been infected with the human immunodeficiency virus (HIV) but who remain clinically well is unknown. Almost certainly the figure is considerably greater than those with AIDS.

The pattern of HIV disease in Europe has closely followed that of the US, with most cases occurring in homosexual and bi-sexual men. In Africa the disease has occurred predominantly in heterosexuals. Recently in Europe increasing numbers of patients who are intravenous drug users with HIV infection have been reported (Box 5.1).

The progressive reduction in cell mediated immunity caused by HIV infection renders the patient vulnerable to a variety of infections. The earliest infections arising as a consequence of impaired cell mediated immunity include bacterial infection particularly with capsulated organisms and also mycobacterium tuberculosis.

A multi-centre study from America early in the AIDS epidemic showed that overall the commonest respiratory infection was *Pneumocystis carinii* pneumonia (PCP) which occurred in about 85% of patients. This was followed by infection with cytomegalovirus (CMV) in approximately 15% of patients, infection with *Mycobacterium avium intracellulare* (4%), and

---

**Box 5.1    Incidence**

- More than 1 500 000 have the disease
- In USA and Europe most are homosexual or bisexual men
- In Africa most are heterosexual
- Cell mediated immunity fails early

---

*Mycobacterium tuberculosis* (4%) and bacterial infections. Pulmonary Kaposi's sarcoma in this early study occurred in a small percentage of patients.

Since the epidemic has progressed later studies have shown that PCP remains the primary opportunistic infection seen in patients with AIDS in both Europe and North America. It is the AIDS defining diagnosis in approximately 65% of cases and up to 80% of patients will develop PCP at some stage in their disease course. PCP is much less common in Africa; here tuberculosis is the major opportunistic infection. In Europe and North America as patients appear to be living longer with their disease as a consequence of earlier presentation to physicians, effective prophylaxis for PCP and antiretroviral therapy with zidovudine (AZT) an increasing proportion of patients develop cutaneous Kaposi's sarcoma; a proportion of these patients also develop pulmonary Kaposi's sarcoma.

## TESTS USED FOR THE DIAGNOSIS OF PULMONARY DISEASE IN HIV POSITIVE PATIENTS

### Non-invasive tests

Non-invasive tests include:

- chest radiography
- arterial blood gas tensions
- transcutaneous oximetry
- pulmonary function tests
- nuclear medicine scanning–gallium-67 scans and $^{99m}$ DTPA scanning.

All these non-invasive tests do not provide a specific diagnosis. Their value is in:

1. Determining the presence or absence of pulmonary disease in HIV positive patients with respiratory symptoms.

2. Assessing the disease severity, for example, the degree of hypoxaemia on exercise or the presence of respiratory failure.

3. Determining whether an invasive test is indicated for establishing an aetiological diagnosis.

4. Monitoring disease progress or response to therapy.

## Tests for aetiological diagnosis

Invasive tests which are used to establish an aetiological diagnosis include:

- sputum induction
- fibreoptic bronchoscopy with bronchoalveolar lavage and/or transbronchial lung biopsy
- open-lung biopsy.

As *Pneumocystis carinii* pneumonia is by far the commonest opportunistic infection in HIV positive patients it has been suggested that a specific diagnosis is not necessary in those patients who present with a typical clinical picture of this pneumonia. Typical features of PCP include a cough which is usually unproductive, a sensation of chest tightness on inspiration not due to pleural pain, progressive dyspnoea initially on exertion and no chest signs on examination (Box 5.2) The chest X-ray may be normal or show a fine ground-glass appearance initially in the perihilar region spreading out into the mid and lower zones. Other patients with PCP may present with less typical features; for example, they may have a rather more gradual onset of symptoms, focal signs within the chest or atypical chest X-ray appearances such as mediastinal adenopathy or intrapulmonary nodules, or a lobar distribution of interstitial shadowing. Most centres now consider it appropriate to establish the exact aetiological cause of the pulmonary symptoms in patients known to be HIV positive or from high-risk groups. This is particularly important if, for example PCP is the presenting infection that brings the HIV infection to light; in this case the diagnosis is essential in order that counselling of the patient

---

> **Box 5.2   Some typical features of PCP**
>
> - Unproductive cough
> - Chest tightness
> - Progressive dyspnoea
> - No signs on examination
> - Chest X-ray—normal
>   —fine ground glass shadowing
>   —perihilar spread

can be commenced with confidence. In addition co-infection, for example PCP with *Mycobacterium tuberculosis*, may be confirmed. This co-infection might be missed if no confirmed microbiological diagnosis was made. Furthermore, once suspicious of PCP treatment could be commenced without prejudicing a diagnostic investigation as soon as convenient.

With increasing use of prophylaxis for PCP and use of AZT it is probable that the incidence of PCP itself will decrease and this infection will become less common. In addition, the clinical manifestations of PCP may become modified by prophylactic treatment, also making a firm diagnosis more important.

### Induced sputum

Patients with AIDS and pulmonary symptoms rarely produce sputum spontaneously so that lung washings or tissue are needed to make a diagnosis. The diagnosis of PCP has become possible by cytological examination of samples of sputum induced by the patient inhaling 20 to 30 ml of 3–5% (hypertonic) saline. This is delivered as a fine mist generated by an ultrasonic nebuliser over 10 to 20 minutes. The material coughed up by the patient within the first 10 minutes of saline inhalation is largely from the oropharynx and central airways; this can be discarded. Sputum obtained after a further 10 minutes of inhalation is likely to contain material from the distal airways and alveoli. This material is usually clear, resembling saliva but unlike saliva, gels on cooling. Purulent sputum is unlikely to contain cysts of *Pneumocystis carinii* and suggests a bacterial cause for the pneumonia. The procedure of sputum induction whilst apparently easy to perform requires special equipment and has been more successful in some centres than in others. Other pathogens may also be detected by standard staining procedures applied to samples of induced sputum. These organisms include *Candida albicans*, *Cryptococcus neoformans*, *Histoplasma capsulatum*, CMV and mycobacteria both typical and atypical.

Use of monoclonal antibodies raised against *Pneumocystis carinii* linked to immunofluorescence stains has been shown to increase the diagnostic yield for sputum induction in the diagnosis of *Pneumocystis carinii* pneumonia. In addition, DNA studies using the technique of the polymerase chain reaction to amplify DNA from *Pneumocystis carinii* also increases the diagnostic yield for this infection in induced sputum.

If the sample of induced sputum is negative for respiratory pathogens then a bronchoscopy should be performed, rather than assuming that there is no detectable infection present. Sputum induction is positive in up to 60% of patients in whom a diagnosis of infection is ultimately made.

### Bronchoscopy

Fibreoptic bronchoscopy is well established as a diagnostic tool for a large range of pulmonary disorders and bronchoalveolar lavage and transbronchial biopsy are widely used.

Bronchoalveolar lavage has been shown to have a very high yield for *Pneumocystis carinii* and the additional benefits of a transbronchial biopsy are very small. Bronchoalveolar lavage is usually performed with small aliquots of normal saline, the total volume of up to 180 ml in three to six divided doses is usual and is remarkably safe. Breathless or hypoxaemic patients should receive supplemental oxygen during and after the procedure. Transbronchial biopsy carries a higher risk of complications including pneumothorax and bleeding in HIV positive patients. The risk is particularly magnified in those patients with PCP; the incidence of pneumothorax is up to 20% in some series.

Bronchoalveolar lavage will identify other infections such as Mycobacterium tuberculosis, atypical mycobacterium, CMV and bacteria. It will however not pick up lymphocytic interstitial pneumonitis, which mimics infections in its clinical presentation, or non-specific pneumonitis. These may only be diagnosed by transbronchial biopsy. Omission of the procedure of transbronchial biopsy simplifies and shortens the procedure and eliminates the complications mentioned above. During bronchoscopy Kaposi's sarcoma lesions may be seen in the endobronchial tree. These lesions are either flat, resembling submucosal haemorrhages or raised, violaceous and may partially occlude an airway.

### Open-lung biopsy

This procedure provides a high diagnostic yield in patients with diffuse lung disease. Most centres would proceed to open-lung biopsy in a patient with respiratory symptoms if two bronchoscopies with lavage have failed to reveal a diagnosis or if despite treatment of a confirmed pathogen the patient continues to deteriorate. In some patients with poor arterial blood gases prior to open-lung biopsy it may be necessary to electively ventilate the patient following biopsy.

## THERAPY OF PULMONARY INFECTIONS IN HIV POSITIVE PATIENTS

### Antiretroviral treatment

Zidovudine (azidothimidine or AZT) is the only antiretroviral agent to have been shown unequivocally to influence HIV replication and to affect the clinical course of symptomatic HIV infection. It is a nucleoside analogue that acts as a reverse transcriptase inhibitor and thus serves as a DNA chain terminator. Early placebo controlled studies showed lower mortality and a lower incidence and severity of opportunistic infections in addition to a greater well being

---

> **Box 5.3  Adverse reactions of zidovudine**
> - Nausea, headache, rash, malaise
> - Bone marrow suppression (in 40%)
> - MCV rises
> - Neutropaenia – affects 30%, later in treatment
> - Necrotising myopathy

in patients treated with this drug. The drug has however substantial bone marrow toxicity, especially for the erythroid and myeloid series. Patients who receive zidovudine show a transient rise in CD4 lymphocytes which occurs within one to two months of commencing treatment. Despite continuing treatment with AZT this rise in CD4 count is not sustained. The HIV p24 antigen falls initially on treatment but the levels will subsequently rise despite continuation of therapy. A proportion of patients will develop nausea, headache, rash and general malaise which may persist. The major medium- to long-term toxicity is from bone marrow suppression and this affects up to 40% of patients. Many patients become transfusion dependent. Occasionally red cell aplasia occurs but the commonest haematological abnormality is a rise in the MCV. Neutropaenia may also frequently occur later in the course of treatment and affects up to 30% of patients; it may be severe and leads to increased susceptibility to staphylococcal and also gram-negative infection. In some patients receiving long-term AZT, necrotising myopathy may occur (Box 5.3). The current prescribing policy is to use 250 mg of AZT orally four times a day. The current indications for AZT therapy in symptomatic HIV positive patients are summarised as:

1. Patients with AIDS following opportunistic infections such as PCP
2. Patients with AIDS related complex
3. Patients with AIDS and opportunistic tumours
4. Patients with AIDS and HIV encephalopathy
5. HIV positive patients with HIV associated thrombocytopaenia

6. Asymptomatic HIV positive patients with rapidly falling CD4 counts

### Other antiretroviral strategies

Several other reverse transcriptase inhibitors are being evaluated:

1. Dideoxycytidine (ddC) has shown activity in phase I studies. It is available on a compassionate use basis. Its main side-effect is peripheral neuropathy.

2. Dideoxyinosine (ddI) is also an antiretroviral. Side-effects attributed to the drug include diarrhoea and acute pancreatitis.

## Pneumocystis carinii

The most common opportunistic infection affecting the lungs in HIV positive patients is PCP. Patients with a CD4 count of $< 200/mm^3$ are at a greatly increased risk of developing this infection. The mortality from the first episode of PCP is now less than 5% but in those patients presenting with PCP who are in respiratory failure the mortality remains over 70%. Primary prophylaxis is given to patients with low CD4 counts in order to prevent the first episode of pneumocystis pneumonia, secondary prophylaxis is given to those patients regardless of CD4 counts who have had one episode of PCP in order to prevent relapse.

In patients presenting with pneumocystis pneumonia there are several clinical features that determine a poor prognosis. These include:

- duration of symptoms of cough and dyspnoea for more than three weeks
- previous episodes of PCP
- extensive radiological shadowing
- hypoxaemia
- elevated serum lactate dehydrogenase enzyme levels
- low serum albumin
- co-infection with other pulmonary pathogens
- extensive interstitial oedema seen on transbronchial lung biopsy specimens

### Treatment of Pneumocystis carinii pneumonia (Box 5.4)

*Co-trimoxazole (trimethoprim and sulphamethoxazole).* This is the best first-line treatment for PCP. High doses of trimethoprim (20 mg/kg/d) and sulphamethoxazole (100 mg/kg/d) in divided doses are used. This regime will generally result in serum concentrations of trimethoprim between 5 and 8 mg/l and is associated with a successful outcome in over 80% of patients who complete therapy. Drug induced neutropaenia is often associated with serum trimethoprim levels up above 25 mg/l. Adjusting the dose of co-trimoxazole to maintain trimethoprim levels between 5 and 8 mg/l considerably reduces haematological toxicity. Most centres will not have facilities for monitoring trimethoprim levels so reductions in the dose of drug to 15 mg/kg/d of trimethoprim and 75 mg/kg of sulphamethoxazole should be carried out if haematological toxicity occurs. Prolonged therapy with co-trimoxazole for between 17 and 21 days is recommended to eradicate infection and reduce the risk of early

---

**Box 5.4   Treatment of PCP**

*Co-trimoxazole* 1st choice
- Trimethoprim 20/mg/kg/day and Sulphamethoxazole 100 mg/kg/day
- Treat for 17–21 days
- At least 10 days of i.v. therapy then oral

Adverse reactions:
- Anorexia, nausea
- Erythrodema and hypersensitivity reactions
- Fever
- Tremor
- Leuco (neutro) penia

*Pentamidine* 2nd choice
- 4 mg/kg/day for 14–21 days
- Painful given i.m.

Adverse reactions:
- Frequent – in 50% of patients
- Hypotension, tachycardia, vomiting
- Flushing, rash, hallucinations
- Thrombocytopaenia
- Hypoglycaemia
- Renal dysfunction – with prolonged use

relapse of infection. Co-trimoxazole is usually given intravenously but is very well absorbed from the gastrointestinal tract. Many centres routinely begin treatment with intravenous co-trimoxazole and as symptoms improve switch to oral treatment at 10 to 14 days to complete therapy. In practice gastrointestinal intolerance is probably all that prevents oral therapy being used routinely in that majority of patients with mild to moderate PCP. In HIV positive patients with PCP adverse reactions to co-trimoxazole have been reported in up to 80% of patients. The cause of this high rate of adverse reactions is unknown but may in part reflect the much higher doses of co-trimoxazole that are used. Common reactions include anorexia, nausea, vomiting, skin rashes including erythro derma, and fever. Nausea and vomiting can usually be controlled with antiemetics. Skin rashes are common, usually mild and rarely progress to exfoliative dermatitis or Stevens–Johnson syndrome. Hypersensitivity reactions with fever and a measles-like rashes will gradually subside despite continued treatment and may be made more tolerable for the patient by giving paracetamol and an antihistamine. Tremor may occur at seven to ten days of treatment; reducing the dose of co-trimoxazole is not usually of benefit and therapy has to be discontinued.

*Pentamidine.* This drug is ineffective orally and is given parenterally. It is usually given in a dose of 4 mg/kg/day for 14 to 21 days. The drug accumulates extensively in body tissues, less than 5% of the drug is excreted unchanged into the urine and the drug may be detected in the urine for six to eight weeks after completion of therapy. Dose reduction of pentamidine during treatment may reduce the frequency and severity of adverse reactions; however, dose reduction may be associated with a poorer outcome from treatment. Intramuscular injection of pentamidine produces considerable local pain, swelling, paraesthesia and myositis, therefore intravenous infusion of pentamidine over one to two hours to avoid hypotension is the preferred route of administration. Pentamidine should not be given intramuscularly.

Adverse reactions to pentamidine occur frequently in up 50% of treated patients and may be severe. Side-effects include hypotension, tachycardia, nausea, vomiting, flushing, rash, hallucinations, altered taste, thrombocytopenia, elevation of liver transaminases. Abnormal glucose metabolism has been noted and hypoglycaemia has been seen as early as two hours after the first infusion but more commonly occurs after seven to ten days of therapy. Persistent hypoglycaemia has also been reported and may continue for several days after discontinuing treatment. Hyperglycaemia has also been described and may require long-term administration of insulin. Pentamidine is directly toxic to β cells in the Islets of Langhans in the pancreas and this results initially in an increased insulin secretion; subsequently the islet cells die and there is dysglycaemia. Renal dysfunction with raised creatinine and urea is the commonest toxicity seen with prolonged therapy, although usually mild; severe renal impairment with death has been reported.

*Co-trimoxazole versus pentamidine.* Both drugs appear equally effective in treating PCP with up to 85% of patients responding to either treatment. Patients normally improve by day five of treatment, somewhat more slowly than with bacterial pneumonia. Defervescence of fever, improved arterial oxygenation and reduction in dyspnoea will have occurred in the majority of patients by day seven of therapy. Improvements in the chest X-ray are often delayed and may take two or three weeks. In comparative studies patients receiving co-trimoxazole responded more rapidly than those receiving pentamidine. Adverse reactions in the two treatment groups occurred with similar frequency. In the clinical setting, patients who failed to respond after five to seven days of treatment with co-trimoxazole or pentamidine are often empirically switched to a new form of treatment. There are no data to show that patients who receive co-trimoxazole and are switched to pentamidine receive any benefit from this.

*Dapsone and trimethoprim.* The combination of dapsone 100 mg/day and trimethoprim 20 mg/kg/day is effective in treating PCP. Common adverse reactions include nausea, vomiting, skin rash, fever, anaemia, neutropaenia and hepatotoxicity. Haemolytic anaemia and methaemoglobinaemia have been described in patients with G6PD deficiency.

*Co-trimoxazole versus dapsone and trimethoprim.* A comparative study of these two regimes showed that oral dapsone and trimethoprim and co-trimoxazole were equally effective in the treatment of PCP but that dapsone and trimethoprim had fewer side-effects.

*Trimetrexate.* This drug is a potent inhibitor of the dehydrofolate reductase system of *Pneumocystis carinii* and is passively taken up and concentrated by protozoal cells. The major side-effect is myelotoxicity and so the drug is given with folinic acid. In patients who failed to respond to first-line treatment with co-trimoxazole and/or pentamidine, trimetrexate used as salvage therapy is effective in up to 70% of patients. Unfortunately, there is a high early relapse rate following treatment with this drug.

*Eflornithine (DFMO).* Eflornithine, which inhibits protozoal ornithine decarboxylase, has also been used in salvage studies in patients with PCP who failed to respond to initial therapy. Used in this context the drug is effective in up to 65% of patients and the main adverse reactions seen include haematological toxicity usually thrombocytopaenia, diarrhoea, reversible hearing loss and alopecia.

*Clindamycin and primaquine.* The combination of clindamycin 600 mg four times daily intravenously and primaquine 15 mg orally daily for 21 days has been shown to be effective in patients who are unresponsive or intolerant of pentamidine and/or co-trimoxazole. Most patients receiving this drug regime develop a macular papular rash despite a good clinical and radiological response.

*Nebulised pentamidine.* Because of the frequent higher rate of adverse reactions to both co-trimoxazole and pentamidine, nebulised delivery of pentamidine has been tried. This delivery method has the potential benefit of both being effective and well tolerated because of the intra-alveolar location of the organism and the limited systemic absorption of the drug. Adequate deposition of pentamidine is dependent on several factors including the droplet size of the aerosol, concentration of drug in the aerosol and the breathing pattern of the patient. The optimal droplet size for maximal alveolar deposition is approximately 2 $\mu$m. Most jet or ultrasonic type nebulisers produce droplets larger than this and so the nebuliser system most frequently used is the Respirgard II (Marquest, Colorado, USA) which is a jet nebuliser and contains baffles to limit the passage of large droplets. Treatment of PCP using inhaled pentamidine involves a once daily inhalation of 600 mg of pentamidine given via the Respirgard nebuliser for 21 days. Several studies have shown that this delivery system and dose of drug is effective in the treatment of patients with mild to moderate PCP. Adverse reactions include cough and bronchoconstriction. Both of these side-effects are alleviated if the patient discontinues smoking during treatment; inhaled $\beta_2$-agonists may be necessary. Hyper-salivation and a metallic taste may also occur.

*New drugs.* BW566 is a 1-4 hydroxynaphthoquinonone with broad spectrum antiprotozoal activity. The drug was originally developed as an antimalarial agent and has been shown to be a selective inhibitor of the mitochondrial electron transport chain in a variety of parasitic protozoa. The site of action appears to be the cytochrome complex of dyhydroorate dehydrogenase, a key enzyme of the pyrimidine biosynthesis pathway. Inhibition of electron transport by hydroxynaphthoquinonone results in the inhibition of pyrimidine biosynthesis. Mammals are able to salvage preformed pyrimidines whereas *Pneumocystis* and other protozoa are unable to do so. This drug has shown activity against PCP in rat and human. Adverse reactions include rash and fever.

*Glucocorticoid therapy.* Despite treatment for PCP some patients deteriorate and develop respiratory failure. The mortality rate is increased in this group. The administration of cortico-steroids in addition to specific antipneumocystis therapy in this patient group has shown to be beneficial. The early additional use of steroid therapy in patients with moderate to severe *Pneumocystis carinii* pneumonia decreases the number requiring ventilatory support and may also improve long-term exercise tolerance. The effects of giving steroids on long-term survival, HIV expression and other unrecognised opportunistic infections is unknown. Until some of these effects are clarified the routine administration of corticosteroids in PCP should be confined to those with moderate to severe pneumonia who are deteriorating despite conventional therapy.

In patients presenting with severe pneumonia or in those who deteriorate despite treatment the diagnosis should be reviewed and further investigations considered.

### Causes of deterioration in patients with Pneumocystis carinii pneumonia

- Severe progressive PCP
- Severe drug side-effects
- Wrong diagnosis (e.g. staphylococcal pneumonia or intrapulmonary Kaposi's sarcoma)
- Co-pathogen infection (e.g. mycobacteria as well as *Pneumocystis carinii*)
- Other complications — pneumothorax
  - left ventricular failure
  - anaemia

The therapeutic options in deteriorating patients are summarised as:

- Consider repeating bronchoscopy or go to open lung biopsy, i.e. is the diagnosis correct?
- Consider treating co-pathogen, e.g. staphylococcus, tuberculosis.
- If treatment is by nebulised pentamidine, change to i.v. high-dose co-trimoxazole or
- If treatment is high-dose i.v. co-trimoxazole, change to i.v. pentamidine
  or eflornithine
  or trimetrexate       } salvage
  or dapsone/pyrimethamine } treatment

or continue i.v. co-trimoxazole and add pulses of methylprednisolone.
- Give supplemental oxygen as required.
- Consider continuous positive airway pressure (CPAP) or intermittent positive pressure ventilation (IPPV).

*Continuous positive airways pressure.* Continuous positive airways pressure ventilation provides positive end expiratory pressure (PEEP) to the airways without the need for intubation.

CPAP is administered via a tight-fitting facial or nasal mask and appears to hold open highly compliant narrow airways throughout the respiratory cycle. Most patients who are hypoxaemic with PCP tolerate CPAP well, and in many patients it maintains or improves arterial oxygen values. Use of CPAP in patients who are deteriorating and becoming hypoxaemic may 'buy valuable time' to allow antimicrobial drugs to work. CPAP is also used in an attempt to avoid intubation and mechanical ventilation.

### General measures in AIDS patients with severe pneumonia

Patients with severe pneumonia who are hypoxaemic should be given supplemental oxygen and fluid replacement as necessary. The volume of fluid required to give intravenous co-trimoxazole needs to be monitored as this may exacerbate the pulmonary fluid overload. The routine use of two litres of normal saline per day should be avoided in this situation and the co-trimoxazole should be diluted in 5% dextrose in water.

### Bacterial infections (Box 5.5)

Patients infected with HIV have a higher incidence of bacterial pneumonia than the normal population. The HIV virus affects T helper (CD4) cell function before CD4 cell numbers fall. This renders patients increasingly susceptible to bacterial infection because opsonisation requires T helper cells to stimulate the B cell activity in order to produce immunoglobulin. In addition, some patients show a selective immunoglobulin G2 sub-class deficiency. The majority of pulmonary bacterial infections respond to broad spectrum antibiotics such as amoxycillin and erythromycin given in conventional doses. Sputum culture in HIV positive patients presenting with bronchitis or pneumonia often reveal *Streptococcus pneumoniae*, *Haemophilus influenzae* and occasionally *Branhamella catarrhalis*. Severe bacterial pneumonia due to *Staphylococcus aureus* or to gram-negative organisms may be seen in patients with the later stages of HIV infection, particularly those patients who are neutropaenic either from HIV infection or from treatment with chemotherapy or ganciclovir for CMV infection.

## Mycobacterial infections (Box 5.6)

Infection with both *Mycobacterium tuberculosis* and atypical mycobacteria is seen with increased frequency in patients who are HIV positive. Tuberculosis may be the first serious infection seen in HIV positive patients and extra pulmonary tuberculosis is now an AIDS defining diagnosis. Patients with tuberculosis who are HIV positive frequently have a negative tuberculin skin test which is in reality a false negative and is caused by anergy. Patients with relatively preserved immune systems and tuberculosis present with a clinical disease pattern similar to the immune competent population. More advanced HIV disease is associated with tuberculosis presenting with atypical infection and a high proportion have disseminated infection. Treatment is with conventional antituberculous therapy. There is a higher rate of

adverse reactions to treatment and it is recommended that treatment is continued for six months after the last documented culture positive result. Following treatment life time secondary prophylaxis with isoniazid is recommended.

Infection with *Mycobacterium avium intracellulare* occurs in advanced HIV disease. The median CD4 is less than 70. This infection occurs in approximately 20% of patients prior to death. It is now well documented that although this infection occurs in end stage HIV disease, it actively contributes to deterioration in patients. *Mycobacterium avium intracellulare* is resistant to conventional first-line antituberculous drugs. Two combination regimes of chemotherapy that have been employed with variable success include amikacin plus ciprafloxacin plus rifampicin plus ethambutol or rifabutin plus chlofazamine plus ciprafloxacin plus ethambutol.

## Cytomegalovirus infection

CMV infection in HIV positive patients occurs in those with profoundly reduced immune indices. CMV may cause a variety of problems outside the thorax including choroidoretinitis, colitis, hepatitis, polyradiculopathy and oesophagitis. In HIV positive patients presenting with respiratory episodes, demonstration of CMV inclusion bodies is not an infrequent finding in patients with other pathologies such as bacterial pneumonia or PCP. It is now well established that treatment of the primary pathogen, either the PCP or bacterial pneumonia, is associated with a good clinical outcome and specific anti CMV treatment is not neces-

---

**Box 5.5   Bacterial infections**

Include:
  *Streptococcus pneumoniae*
  *Haemophilus influenzae*
  *Staphylococcus aureus*
  *Gram-negative bacilli*
  *Branhamella catarrhalis*
Most respond to broad spectrum antibiotics

---

**Box 5.6   Mycobacterial infections**

• Increasingly common. Not only in Africa
• May be the first serious AIDS related infection
• Tuberculin test often negative
• Many present with disseminated infection
• High rate of adverse reactions to treatment
• Life-time secondary prophylaxis is recommended

sary. Rarely CMV is pathogenic in the lung and is associated with a pneumonitis similar to that seen in patients with allogenic renal, liver, heart or bone marrow transplants. In this situation treatment is with intravenous ganciclovir at a dose of 10 mg/kg/day given for three weeks. Maintenance therapy may be required thereafter on an indefinite basis to prevent relapse.

*Kaposi's sarcoma.* In addition to causing cutaneous lesions, Kaposi's sarcoma may involve parenchymal structures. Within the thorax Kaposi's sarcoma may involve the pleura, the parenchyma of the lungs, lymph nodes or the bronchial tree. When significant pleuro- pulmonary disease is present there is invariably extensive evidence of Kaposi's sarcoma at other sites, particularly the skin and the palate. Endobronchial lesions may progress to produce obstruction, and pleural effusions are particularly troublesome and recur despite aspiration and pleurodesis. Radiotherapy may be given to treat tracheal or proximal bronchial lesions or chemotherapy with bleomycin may be used to treat parenchymal disease producing dyspnoea or haemoptysis (Box 5.7).

### Prevention of lung infections

*Prophylaxis of PCP.* PCP occurs most commonly in immunosuppressed individuals with median and CD4 counts of 100/mm³. When the CD4 count is less than 200/mm³ patients have a 70% chance of developing PCP in the ensuing 18 months. There is a clear need for primary prophylaxis in such patients. In addition, primary prophylaxis is also recommended for any patient who has an AIDs defining diagnosis regardless of their CD4 count, for example, patients with toxoplasmosis, lymphoma or Kaposi's sarcoma. Secondary prophylaxis should be given to all patients who have had PCP. Both co-trimoxazole and pentamidine given either once monthly via a nebuliser or intermittently by the intravenous route are shown to be effective. Randomised trials comparing co-trimoxa-

---

**Box 5.7    Respiratory infections**

PCP in 85% of cases
CMV (15%)
Mycobacterium avium intracellulare (4%)
MTB (4%)
Kaposi's sarcoma (2%)

NB. TB is the commonest infection in African patients. Infections may co-exist.

---

zole by mouth with nebulised pentamidine show that co-trimoxazole is more effective. Ideally prophylactic treatment should be cheap, easy to take and have no toxic side-effects. Co-trimoxazole fulfils this role but produces a skin rash in some patients. Side-effects are less frequent when the dose is 960 mg daily or given on alternate days. Nebulised pentamidine is expensive and effective but not easy to take. Current recommendations are to use 300 mg of pentamidine via a Respirgard II nebuliser given once monthly. Non-comparative studies have shown that daily dapsone, with or without weekly pyrimethamine and sulphadoxine with pyrimethamine (fansidar) are possible alternatives for prophylaxis. Most centres now routinely offer prophylaxis with oral co-trimoxazole 960 mg once daily or on alternate days for both primary and secondary prophylaxis of PCP. If this is not tolerated, monthly nebulised pentamidine is used. If both methods are unacceptable, dapsone 50 mg daily is an acceptable alternative.

*Prevention of tuberculosis.* Tuberculosis arises due to endogenous reactivation of latent infection. It is suggested that patients who are both HIV and tuberculin skin test positive will develop tuberculosis. However, in a study in which isoniazid prophylaxis was given no patient developed tuberculosis. The efficacy of isoniazid as preventative treatment in patients with HIV has not been formally evaluated. It is likely to be highly effective against tuberculosis in HIV positive patients.

*Prevention of bacterial pneumonia.* Despite the high incidence of bacterial infections in patients with AIDS there is no good evidence that preventative measures exist. HIV infection diminishes the patient's antibody response to capsular polysaccharide vaccines used for the prophylaxis of pneumococcal pneumonia.

## FURTHER READING

Miller R F, Mitchell D M 1992 Pneumocystis carinii pneumonia: AIDS and the lung – update 92. Thorax 47: 305–314

Mitchell D, Woodcock A (eds) 1990 AIDS and the lung. BMA Publications, London

Mitchell D M, Miller R F 1992 Respiratory complications of HIV disease. AIDS and the lung–update 92. Thorax 47: 381–390

CHAPTER CONTENTS

**Epidemiology   97**

**Drugs used in treatment   98**
Rifampicin   98
Isoniazid   101
Ethambutol   102
Streptomycin   102
Pyrazinamide   103
Thiacetazone   103
PAS   104
Cycloserine   105
Prothionamide and ethionamide   105
Capreomycin   105
New drugs   105

**Generalised reactions to antituberculous
drugs   106**
Cutaneous and generalised hypersensitivity
reactions   106
 Management   106
Hepatitis   106

**Drug regimens   106**
Newly diagnosed patients   107
Fully supervised intermittent regimens   108
Less potent regimens   108

**Drugs in special situations   109**
Renal impairment   109
Liver impairment   110
Pregnancy   110
Tuberculous meningitis   110
Tuberculosis in immunosuppressed patients   111

**Chemotherapy in extrapulmonary tuberculosis   111**
Treatment of the primary lesion   111
Tuberculous pericarditis   112
Tuberculous laryngitis   112

**Atypical mycobacterial infections   112**

**Management when primary chemotherapy has
failed   112**

**Chemoprophylaxis   113**

# 6

# Tuberculosis

## EPIDEMIOLOGY

The epidemiology of tuberculosis differs greatly between technically advanced and developing countries. Eradication of tuberculosis even in the technically advanced countries is unlikely to happen for many years yet; not only is there a potentially large reservoir of infected individuals who may still develop the disease, but also the decline has slowed in many countries because of large-scale immigration from areas of high prevalence.

It is estimated that at the present time there are 8–10 million new cases every year and 3.5 million deaths. In most parts of the Western world tuberculosis has been declining steadily for many years. Concern is growing however about the resurgence of the disease in a number of countries. For example, notifications in England and Wales increased by 8% between 1987 and 1989 (the evidence suggests that HIV infection is not yet directly implicated); in Switzerland the increase was 15% between 1989 and 1990 (due to a large increase in foreigners), and between 1978 and 1991 the proportion of notifications in New York compared with the whole of the US rose from 4.6% to 15.7% (due to deterioration of public health services, socio-economic decline, and impoverishment complicated by the HIV epidemic).

The eradication of tuberculosis has been the goal in technically advanced countries, but in the future the effect of HIV will have a major impact on delaying this target. This is currently more of a problem in developing countries where the association of HIV and tuberculosis is much more prevalent – particularly in Africa. Any reduction in the number of smear positive cases in the developing world would be recognised as a major achievement.

## DRUGS USED IN TREATMENT

The drugs which are most commonly used for previously untreated patients are:

- Rifampicin                  (R)
- Isoniazid                   (H)
- Ethambutol                  (E)
- Pyrazinamide                (Z)
- Streptomycin                (S)
- Thiacetazone                (T)
- Para-aminosalicylic acid    (P)

The usual doses for daily and intermittent regimens are shown in Tables 6.1 and 6.2. If pri-mary treatment fails, second line drugs that can be given include:

- Cycloserine       (CYC)
- Prothionamide     (PRO)
- Ethionamide       (ETH)
- Capreomycin       (CAP)
- Viomycin          (VIO)
- Kanamycin         (KAN)

## Rifampicin

Rifampicin is a broad spectrum antibiotic derived from *Streptomyces mediterranei*, whose in vivo and in vitro activity against *Mycobacterium tuberculosis* was first demonstrated in 1967. It is also effective against staphylococci, strepto-cocci, *Clostridia*, coliforms, *Pseudomonas* spp, *Proteus* spp, *Salmonella*, *Shigella* and *Bacteroides* spp.

Rifampicin (Box 6.1) is almost completely absorbed from the gastrointestinal tract after an

| Table 6.1 Drug doses – daily | | | | |
|---|---|---|---|---|
| Drug | Adults & children mg/kg | Weight | Adults | Dose |
| Rifampicin | 10 | < 50 kg<br>> 50 kg | | 450 mg<br>600 mg |
| Isoniazid | 5 | | | 300 mg |
| Streptomycin | 15–20 (max 1 g) | | | 1 g (< 40 yrs)<br><br>0.75 g (> 40 yrs) |
| Pyrazinamide | 35 | > 50 kg<br>50–74 kg<br><br>< 75 kg | | 1.5 g<br>2.0 g<br><br>2.5 g |
| Ethambutol | 15 | | | |
| Thiacetazone | 4 (for children) | | | 150 mg |
| Para-aminosalicylic acid (PAS) | 300 | | | 10–12 g |

**Box 6.1   Rifampicin**

Absorption: Oral rapid
            Enzyme induced

Bactericidal

Adverse reactions:
        Gastrointestinal, cutaneous
        Hepatitis
        Thrombocytopenia, Flu-syndrome
        'Red-man' syndrome
        Acute haemolytic anaemia

oral dose and is partly deacetylated in the liver by enzymes which are induced in the first few days of treatment. It is excreted almost completely by the bile but 10% is excreted in urine, there being an enterohepatic circulation. When taken on an empty stomach absorption is rapid and peak serum levels – 10 to 12 $\mu$g/ml after 600 mg orally – are reached in two or three hours, some rifampicin still being present after 24 hours. The pharmacokinetic disposal of rifampicin is dose dependent, larger doses resulting in greater than proportional peak serum levels and slower than proportional rates of elimination. The half-life is unaffected by impaired renal function. Rifampicin is found in the CSF at 2 hours and at 6 hours the minimum inhibitory capacity for *Mycobacterium tuberculosis* is achieved. The CSF concentration usually approaches 20% of serum concentration. The concentration in the CSF declines during the course of treatment, probably associated with a lessening of meningeal inflammation as a response to treatment, but therapeutic concentrations can be maintained during the first two months of treatment. Ideally the drug should be administered once a day, preferably, but not essentially, less than half an hour before breakfast. If nausea and vomiting are a problem, administration last thing at night is advised. The dose may need to be reduced in the presence of liver disease and in the elderly.

It is sometimes necessary to give the drug intravenously. A 600 mg vial of powdered

**Table 6.2   Drug dosages– intermittent therapy**

| Drug | Adults & children mg/kg | Weight | Adults Dose |
|---|---|---|---|
| Rifampicin | 15 | | 600–900 mg |
| Isoniazid | 15 | | + 10 mg of pyridoxine |
| Streptomycin | 15–20 | < 50 kg > 50 kg | 750mg 1 g |
| Pyrazinamide | 50 three times a week | < 50 kg | 2 g |
| | 75 two times a week | > 50 kg | 2.5 g |
| Ethambutol | 30 three times a week | < 50 kg | 3 g |
| | 45 two times a week | > 50 kg | 3.5 g |

rifampicin is reconstituted with 10 ml of solvent solution and immediately diluted with 500 ml of infusion fluid. The infusion takes 2 to 3 hours.

### Adverse reactions

Adverse reactions to daily rifampicin are rarely serious but when serious toxicity does occur it is often discovered that the patient has been taking the drug intermittently through non-compliance or has recommenced treatment after an interval. All patients should be warned to expect that the urine, sweat and tears will be coloured pink.

*Gastrointestinal reactions* – nausea, anorexia, mild abdominal pain are the most common, vomiting and diarrhoea occur less frequently. These reactions occur in less than 5% of patients and are commoner in the elderly. They can be overcome by administering a smaller dose for three or four days or by giving the drug at night. Sometimes administration during a meal can solve the problem.

*Cutaneous reactions* – usually mild and consist of flushing of the skin sometimes accompanied by itchiness and occasionally by a rash. The reaction comes on two to three hours after taking the drug and lasts for several hours and begins early in treatment. The patients usually desensitise themselves. More serious generalised cutaneous reactions can occur as with other anti-tuberculous drugs (see Section 3).

*Hepatitis* during rifampicin administration among patients with no history of liver disease or of alcoholism is small. The addition of isoniazid and pyrazinamide does not appear to increase the risk of hepatitis. Alcoholism is not a contraindication to the use of rifampicin plus isoniazid containing regimens but it is suggested that in patients with cirrhosis, bilirubin concentrations greater than 50 $\mu$mol/l should be an indication for reduction in rifampicin dose. Transient rise in hepatic enzymes is commonly observed in the early weeks of treatment but monitoring of liver function is necessary only in alcoholics and patients with impaired liver function.

*Thrombocytopaenic purpura* sometimes occurs in patients on daily treatment.

*Rarer problems* – osteomalacia, pseudomembranous colitis and pseudo-adrenal crises have been described in association with rifampicin. If the latter event is suspected, urgent treatment with corticosteroids should be given. Poisoning due to an overdose of rifampicin results in the 'red man' syndrome which may be fatal. The skin and subsequently the sclera become reddish-orange in colour; nausea, vomiting, abdominal pain and convulsions have been observed. Treatment is supportive.

*Adverse reactions with intermittent rifampicin:*

The flu syndrome is characterised by fever, shivering and malaise with headache, dizziness and bone pain occasionally. The symptoms develop shortly after taking the drug and last for up to 8 hours. This is often self-limiting. Management if necessary is by reducing the dose size or changing temporarily to a daily regimen. Syndromes associated with thrombocytopaenia and purpura are very rare on daily treatment but with intermittent treatment the thrombocytopaenia can be extreme and the drug should be stopped at once and never repeated.

Acute haemolytic anaemia – systemic symptoms and acute haemolysis can occur within a few hours of a dose and there is a danger of development of renal failure. Rifampicin dependent antibodies are found in the serum. Acute renal failure can occasionally develop.

Mild eosinophilia has occasionally been reported but is of no significance.

Rifampicin is a potent inducer of liver enzymes which may increase the metabolism of certain other drugs being administered concomitantly. The most important are corticosteroids, oestrogens including the oral contraceptive pill, oral coumarin anticoagulants, oral diabetic agents, digoxin, methadone, morphine, dapsone, ketoconazole and cyclosporin. Patients requiring rifampicin and using the oral contraceptive pill should be advised to take an alternative method of contraception.

When resuming treatment with rifampicin after a prolonged interval the drug should be given in small gradually increasing doses. The initial adult dose should be 150 mg daily and the dose increased by 150 mg per day until the full dose is given. Renal function and platelet function should be monitored during this period.

## Isoniazid

Isoniazid (Box 6.2) is isonicotinyl hydrazine, a chemical identified to be active against mycobacteria in 1952. Its important assets are its potency, its rare toxicity and its low cost. Isoniazid when given orally is readily absorbed. There is good distribution throughout the tissues and therapeutic levels are obtained in the cerebrospinal fluid, lung cavities and caseous material. There is no cross resistance with other mycobacterial drugs. The drug is not protein bound. The peak serum concentrations are obtained within 1 to 3 hours but effective levels are still present 24 hours later. Some of the drug is excreted in the urine unchanged but a proportion is altered metabolically, mostly by acetylation in the liver by the substance acetyltransferase. The acetylated derivative is almost devoid of antibacterial activity. The degree of conversion to an inactive form is fairly constant for any one individual. There are however genetically determined variations in the rate of acetylation. In some ethnic groups the frequency of rapid inactivation is high. Thus the Japanese, Koreans and in particular the Eskimos have a prevalence of rapid inactivators ranging from 50 to 95% whereas in South India it is about 5%. Europeans are predominantly slow inactivators. In slow acetylators the concentrations of free drug in the urine and serum are higher. The mean serum half lives are about 1.4 hours for rapid acetylators and 3 hours for slow acetylators. There is now a relatively simple urine test available for phenotyping isoniazid inactivators.

The drug is usually given orally once daily but in the treatment of meningitis is sometimes given in solution intrathecally. It is also available intravenously and intramuscularly. The recommended standard oral daily dose is 300 mg or 5 mg/kg body weight, this being adequate in clinical practice even in rapid acetylators.

### Adverse reactions

Generalised cutaneous reactions are much less frequently caused by isoniazid than by rifampicin, PAS or streptomycin.

Hepatitis may occasionally be severe but is most common (2%) when the drug is used chemoprophylactically in adults over the age of 35.

Peripheral neuropathy is the main form of chronic toxicity. Other less common forms of neurological disturbances are optic neuritis, toxic psychosis, generalised convulsions, difficulty with micturition, tremor and hyper-reflexia.

Peripheral neuropathy is very uncommon in well-nourished patients treated with recommended doses. It is more likely to occur in malnourished patients where high doses are employed and in slow acetylators of the drug. Others at risk include the elderly, patients with chronic liver disease, alcoholics and pregnant women. The neuropathy can be prevented by the simultaneous administration of pyridoxine 10 mg daily. Higher doses of pyridoxine may interfere with the antibacterial activity of isoniazid.

Pellagra has been produced by the exacerbation of niacin deficiency by isoniazid in undernourished individuals.

---

Box 6.2   Isoniazid

Cheap
Absorption:        Oral, rapid

Fast and slow acetylators

Adverse reactions:        Hepatitis
                          Peripheral neuropathy
                          Pellagra

Other rare reactions are haemolytic anaemia in patients with glucose 6-phosphate dehydrogenase deficiency, agranulocytosis, lupoid reactions and arthralgia. Isoniazid is not harmful in pregnancy.

## Ethambutol

Ethambutol is a synthetic compound unrelated to previous antituberculous drugs. It is active against *Mycobacterium tuberculosis* and in addition against some strains of photocromogens, e.g. *Mycobacterium kansasii*. It is water soluble and easily absorbed. Its action is bacteriostatic and for therapeutic efficacy serum levels of 3 to 5 $\mu$g/ml are required and are obtained by a once daily dose of 15 to 25 mg/kg bodyweight. Excretion is mainly by the urine, the drug still being in an active form.

Ethambutol is administered orally (Box 6.3). The larger doses originally employed produced an unacceptable level of adverse effects and are no longer necessary. In short-term chemotherapy for the newly diagnosed patient ethambutol is used as a companion drug to rifampicin and isoniazid, the dose sometimes recommended being 25 mg/kg bodyweight for 2 months and then 15 mg/kg. Most people however now use only 15 mg/kg throughout treatment. Only very rarely indeed is the lower dose responsible for any adverse effects.

### Adverse reactions

Ethambutol is generally well tolerated, its main adverse reaction being retrobulbar neuritis. Retrobulbar neuritis causes reduced visual acuity, central scotoma and disturbance of red/green perception. The occurrence of this side-effect on a daily dose of 15 mg/kg is exceptionally unusual. If 25 mg/kg is given as a starting dose patients should always be told that ethambutol may affect vision and the drug should be stopped immediately should vision become impaired.

Other very uncommon adverse effects are numbness and paraesthesiae of the limbs, arthralgia, hepatitis and peripheral neuropathy. General hypersensitivity reactions are rare.

## Streptomycin

Like isoniazid and rifampicin, streptomycin is bactericidal in action (Box 6.4). As intestinal absorption is negligible the drug must be administered by intramuscular injection. After an injection of 1 g, serum levels of 25 – 50 $\mu$g/ml are obtained, well above the minimal therapeutic level of about 7 $\mu$g/ml. The plasma half life is considerably longer in the new born and in patients over 40 years of age than in other people. The drug diffuses readily into most body tissues but there are only very low concentrations achieved in the CSF. The drug crosses the placenta and fetal serum levels are about half of those in maternal blood. The drug is excreted almost entirely by glomerular filtration and thus it is important to modify dosage in persons who may have impaired renal function. Streptomycin sulphate for intramuscular use is given as a standard adult dose of 1 g in patients below 40 years and between the ages of 40 and 60 years the dose should be reduced to 0.75 g. Above the age of 60 and in patients known to

---

**Box 6.3  Ethambutol**

Bacteriostatic
Administration:        oral
Adverse reactions:     Retrobular neuritis (high-
                       dose therapy only)
                       Numbness and paraesthesia
                       Arthralgia

---

**Box 6.4  Streptomycin**

Bactericidal
Administration:        parenteral
Renally excreted
Adverse reactions:     8th Cranial nerve damage
                       Anaphylaxis
                       Renal damage

have renal impairment, the correct dose should be attained by monitoring serum levels. Wherever possible, one should abandon the use of streptomycin because of the danger of transmission of HIV infection.

### Adverse reactions

Streptomycin has a selective toxic action on the 8th cranial nerve and vestibular damage is very much more common than auditory damage. Vestibular damage is more frequent in older patients and is dose related. It usually occurs within the first 3 months of treatment. Occasionally symptoms have a dramatic onset but more commonly the patient complains of progressive giddiness. Nystagmus may be present. The damage to the nerve is permanent but provided the drug is stopped immediately most patients lose their symptoms in a matter of weeks through compensatory mechanisms. Deafness occurs extremely rarely and usually only in patients whose hearing was already impaired.

Other adverse effects:

- anaphylaxis
- renal damage: like other aminoglycosides streptomycin is potentially nephrotoxic causing proximal tubular damage. Proteinuria, casts and elevated serum urea may be observed.

Streptomycin has been found to potentiate the neuromuscular block produced by curare and is therefore contraindicated in individuals with myasthenia gravis.

Extremely rarely streptomycin has been suggested as the cause of haemolytic anaemia, aplastic anaemia, agranulocytosis, thrombocytopaenia and lupoid reactions. Intrathecal streptomycin may rarely cause root pain, retention of urine and nystagmus.

## Pyrazinamide

Pyrazinamide is a highly bacteriocidal drug which is most effective at a pH of about 5.8 (Box

---

> **Box 6.5   Pyrazinamide**
>
> Bactericidal
> Oral
> Adverse reactions:          Hepatotoxic
>                             Arthralgia
>                             Anaemia
>                             Nausea

---

6.5). Thus it is active against intracellular mycobacteria having a sterilising effect on organisms growing slowly in macrophages. It is very valuable in short course treatment and in tuberculous meningitis. Its antibacterial activity is largely limited to *Mycobacterium tuberculosis*.

The drug is always administered orally. The standard dose for adults and children is 35 mg/kg in an oral dose. If intravenous therapy is present lyophilized morphazinamide is available in 1 g vials.

### Adverse reactions

The commonest adverse effects of pyrazinamide are hepatotoxicity and arthralgia. The hepatotoxicity ranges from mild disturbance of liver function discovered on biochemical tests only, through a syndrome of mild fever, anorexia, tender enlargement of the liver and spleen to more serious reactions including clinical jaundice and occasionally fulminating acute yellow atrophy.

Arthralgia is a relatively frequent reaction and affects both large and small joints. It usually appears in the first 2 months of treatment and is commoner in Chinese. It is due to the inhibition of the renal tubular secretion of uric acid by pyrazinamide.

Cutaneous hypersensitivity reactions are rare. Other rare adverse effects include anorexia, nausea, vomiting and sideroblastic anaemia.

## Thiacetazone

Thiacetazone is rarely used in technically advanced countries but is widely used in developing countries (Box 6.6). It is of low potency but is effective as a companion drug in prevent-

---

Box 6.6   Thiacetazone

Administration: oral
Cheap
Low potency
Adverse reactions:   Cutaneous – exfoliative
                           dermatitis
                       Giddiness
                       Dizziness
                       Anaemia
                       Conjunctivitis
                       Hepatitis

---

ing the development of isoniazid resistance and is a satisfactory substitute for PAS, particularly because of its low cost. It has been shown to be poorly tolerated by the Chinese population of Singapore and Hong Kong, badly tolerated by Caucasians but surprisingly well tolerated in East African countries and in South America. Its advantages over PAS are that the patient needs to swallow only one tablet daily. The drug is stable in tropical countries, keeps well whereas PAS is liable to deteriorate; its cost is one-tenth of that of PAS. Natural resistance to thiacetazone occurs in varying proportions of strains of mycobacteria, being high in Madras, moderately high in Hong Kong, and fairly low in East Africa and in Britain. There may be cross resistance between thiacetazone and ethionamide.

Thiacetazone is administered orally, the normal dose being 150 mg once a day. The dose is crucial as a higher dose greatly increases tox-icity and a lower dose decreases efficacy.

### Adverse reactions

The commonest adverse effect is a generalised cutaneous reaction, exfoliative dermatitis or Stevens–Johnson syndrome. Sometimes very severe giddiness, dizziness or gastrointestinal symptoms can occur.

Other adverse effects, some of which may be serious, include anaemia, agranulocytosis and thrombocytopenia, cerebral oedema, conjunctivitis, blurred vision and jaundice. The drug should not be given to patients with liver dis-

ease or with renal failure because it is excreted partially unchanged by the kidneys.

## Para-aminosalicylic acid (PAS)

PAS was introduced in 1946 and is bacteriostatic (Box 6.7). It is now virtually unobtainable in many countries. Its principal value is as an effective companion drug particularly to isoniazid, preventing the emergence of isoniazid resistant organisms. It does not reach the CSF in therapeutic concentrations. Although in technically advanced countries it is rarely used today, having been replaced by ethambutol and rifampicin, it remains an important drug in developing countries because it is relatively inexpensive and a valuable one in combined regimens. PAS is bulky and unpleasant to take, the cachets being large in size and the tablets numerous. The usual dose is 10 to 12 g daily in 2 divided doses.

### Adverse reactions

Gastrointestinal disturbance and generalised hypersensitivity reactions are the main adverse reactions; hypokalaemia may also occur.

Gastrointestinal disturbance is common. Diarrhoea can be severe and anorexia, nausea, vomiting and abdominal discomfort are more common. Haematological toxicity includes hypoprothrombinaemia, haemolytic anaemia and thrombocytopaenia but these are rare. Acute renal failure is very rare. Prolonged administration of PAS can cause hypothyroidism and goitre as PAS has an antithyroid effect inhibiting the synthesis of thyroxine.

---

Box 6.7   PAS

Bacteriostatic
Administration:          oral (unpleasant)
Adverse reactions:       Gastrointestinal disturbance
                         Rashes
                         Anaemia

---

## Cycloserine

Cycloserine has a relatively weak effect against mycobacteria when given alone but may be valuable in preventing resistance for instance to ethionamide. It is preferably given in triple combination. The drug is given orally. The initial dose being 250 mg 12 hourly increased to 250 mg every 8 hours and if tolerated, a maximum dose of 500 mg every 12 hours.

### Adverse reactions

The main reactions to cycloserine concern the central nervous system causing dizziness, slurred speech, convulsions, headache, insomnia and often severe depression, altered behaviour and occasionally suicide. Generalised reactions and hepatitis are rare. The drug should be avoided in patients with a history of epilepsy, anxiety, psychotic states or alcoholism. There is no information on its safety in pregnancy.

## Prothionamide and ethionamide

Prothionamide while essentially similar to ethionamide in its anti-bacterial effects is considered to be the less unpleasant of the two drugs to take and is tending to replace the latter. The drug is freely distributed throughout the body and reaches the CSF even in healthy individuals.

The drug is usually given as 125 mg tablets with an optimum daily dose of 1 g. The main adverse effects are gastrointestinal with anorexia, nausea and a metallic taste. Psychic disturbances ranging from drowsiness to psychoses, hallucinations and depression have been reported. An important, though very rare reaction, is hypoglycaemia. Control of diabetic patients taking this drug requires particular care. Hepatitis is observed in about 10% of patients but is rarely serious. The drug should not be administered in pregnancy as it has been shown to have teratogenic properties in animals.

## Capreomycin

Capreomycin is an aminoglycoside antibiotic obtained from *Streptomyces capreolus*. Absorption from the gut is poor and the drug must be given intramuscularly. There is no cross resistance between streptomycin and capreomycin. It is given as 1 g intramuscularly daily. The adverse effects are similar to those of streptomycin. Pain and induration at injection sites may also be observed.

## New drugs

There is still a need for highly effective new drugs as there is a need to expand the number of available drugs in the face of increasing resistance to current drugs, to shorten further the period of treatment and to facilitate fully supervised regimens. It is also important to find more effective treatment for the opportunistic mycobacteria especially *Mycobacterium avium intracellulare*.

The new rifamycins may achieve many of these aims. These are more active than quinolones and are only just effective in tuberculosis at current dose level. Of the rifamycins a number of derivatives have been explored including rifapentine, rifabutin and rathadine. Much more knowledge is required before these come into general use but rifabutin may be effective against and of use in some strains resistant to rifampicin.

Fluorinated quinolones such as ciprofloxacin, ofloxacin and difloxacin appear to be only just effective in tuberculosis.

## GENERALISED REACTIONS TO ANTITUBERCULOUS DRUGS

### Cutaneous and generalised hypersensitivity reactions

The clinical manifestations are rash and fever. Fever may be the only manifestation initially and is often confused with the effects of the disease itself. The rash is erythematous and itchy, may be macular or papular and if severe, urticarial. It is most prominent on the face, neck and extremities. It can progress to exfoliative dermatitis and anaphylaxis is another potentially serious adverse event.

### Management

Minor rashes are commonly due to rifampicin and these can be treated with antihistamines. However if the rash progresses the drug should be withdrawn.

Once the reaction has subsided daily challenge doses to the possible offending drug should be given. A possible sequence is shown in Table 6.3. Challenge doses of the drugs in the regimen should be given in the sequence shown as the last three drugs in the table are the most likely to cause a reaction. If the initial generalised reaction was severe then smaller initial challenge doses should be given, approximately one-tenth the dose suggested in Table 6.3 for day 1. If no reaction occurs to the challenge dose the drug may be resumed in full dose though it must be clearly understood that if desensitisation is carried out, this must be done under cover of two antituberculosis drugs to which the patient is not hypersensitive as drug resistance has been described as emerging during desensitisation procedures when this precaution was not observed.

In most patients desensitisation is easily achieved. If reaction occurs to the first challenge dose, one-tenth of this dose should be given as the initial desensitising dose and the dose doubled each day until full dosage is achieved.

In patients who have severe reactions, except those who have had exfoliative dermatitis in whom desensitisation should never be attempted, the procedure can be carried out under corticosteroid cover.

## Hepatitis

Hepatitis can be caused by all antituberculous drugs although it is rarely due to ethambutol or cycloserine. It may be difficult to decide

**Table 6.3  Challenge doses for detecting cutaneous or generalised hypersensitivity to antituberculous drugs**

| Drug | Challenge Day 1 | Doses Day 2 |
|---|---|---|
| Isoniazid | 50 mg | 300 mg |
| Rifampicin | 75 mg | 300 mg |
| Pyrazinamide | 250 mg | 1.0 g |
| Ethionamide, prothionamide | 125 mg | 375 mg |
| Cycloserine | 125 mg | 250 mg |
| Ethambutol | 100 mg | 500 mg |
| Para-aminosalicylic acid | 1.0 g | 5.0 g |
| Thiacetazone | 25 mg | 50 mg |
| Streptomycin or other aminoglycosides | 125 mg | 500 mg |

Reproduced with permission from Horne N W 1990 Modern drug treatment of tuberculosis. The data are from Girling D J 1982 Adverse effects of antituberculous drugs. Drugs 23: 56–74.

whether hepatitis occurring in any patient is due to drug treatment and if due to drug toxicity, which drugs are responsible. The frequency of hepatitis as an adverse effect of antituberculosis therapy is low with large studies analysed from all over the world suggesting an incidence of zero to 5%. Isoniazid when used alone as chemoprophylaxis has in some series been associated with a frequency of hepatitis at a risk of 5/1000 subjects, the risk increasing with age. It is suggested therefore that isoniazid chemoprophylaxis should be avoided whenever possible in adults over the age of 35. With modern pyrazinamide regimens (the incidence of hepatitis was high when 40 to 50 mg/kg bodyweight doses were used) there does not appear to be a high incidence of hepatitis – the frequency being 0.2–2.8%.

## DRUG REGIMENS

The aims of chemotherapy are:

- to cure patients with minimum interference with their lives

- to prevent death from active disease or its late effects
- to avoid relapse
- to prevent emergence of acquired resistance
- to protect the community from infection

With the modern chemotherapeutic drugs it is now possible to induce bactericidal treatment to rapidly minimise the risk of further infection and contamination. This has had the effect of significantly reducing the spread of disease to contacts. Intensive bactericidal drug treatment also minimises the probability of new and resistant mutants appearing and there is less likelihood of the emergence of 'persisters'. The initial modern intensive phase of chemotherapy is therefore of tremendous importance. The drugs which are most commonly used are rifampicin, isoniazid, streptomycin, pyrazinamide and ethambutol, the latter probably contributing nothing to sterilising activity but being of value in preventing the emergence of drug resistant strains.

The antituberculous drugs vary in:

- their bactericidal action, defined as their ability to kill large numbers of actively metabolising bacilli rapidly;
- their sterilising action, defined as their capacity to kill special populations of slowly or intermittently metabolising semi-dormant bacilli: the so-called 'persisters';
- their ability to prevent the emergence of acquired resistance by suppressing drug resistant mutants present in all large bacterial populations;
- their suitability for intermittent use.

*Bactericidal action.* Most of the antituberculosis drugs with the exception of thiacetazone and PAS have some bactericidal action, but isoniazid is the most potent bactericidal drug. It may kill some 90% of the bacilliary population within the first few days of chemotherapy. Rifampicin is also an important bactericidal drug with streptomycin and pyrazinamide being less potent.

*Sterilising action.* Rifampicin and pyrazinamide are the most important drugs here because of their ability to kill semi-dormant bacilli capable of surviving the bactericidal action of isoniazid and so giving risk to relapse after treatment.

*Preventing the emergence of acquired resistance.* Even populations which have not been exposed to antituberculosis drugs contain small proportions of drug resistant mutants. Isoniazid and rifampicin are the most effective at preventing emergence of resistance to other drugs and streptomycin and ethambutol are only slightly less so.

*Suitability for intermittent use.* Isoniazid, rifampicin, pyrazinamide, streptomycin and ethambutol are all effective when given 3 times or twice a week.

When the total duration of treatment is reduced which is the main advantage of short course therapy, a smaller total quantity of drug is required which makes the cost less. Furthermore the strain placed on patients who have to take drugs for a long period is reduced and therefore compliance likely to be increased and default decreased. The shorter period of treatment with less supervision is likely to have an input in terms of cost, facilities and health personnel. Of great importance is that due to the initial intensive phase killing off tubercle bacilli rapidly: patients are less likely to relapse if they default, and if they do relapse they do so with sensitive organisms.

## Newly diagnosed patients

The regimen should include the main sterilising drugs and the above 6-month regimen is recommended (Table 6.4) (2HRZ/4HR – note the duration of treatment in months is given as a figure before the initials of each drug combination. A subset figure e.g. $_2$ or $_3$ indicates a twice- or thrice-weekly regimen.)

The above regimen should achieve a 100% cure in patients who comply and in whom the organisms are initially sensitive.

| Table 6.4 | Recommended 6-month regimen | |
|---|---|---|
| Isoniazid | 300 mg orally | |
| Rifampicin | 600 mg (> 50 kg) | for 6 months/daily |
| | 450 mg (< 50 kg) | |
| Pyrazinamide | 1.5 g (< 50 kg) | |
| | 2.0 g (50 –74 kg) | for initial 2 months/daily |
| | 2.5 g (> 75 kg) | |
| Some physicians choose to add: | | |
| Ethambutol | 15–25 mg/kg orally | |
| | (see text) | for initial 2 months/daily |
| Streptomycin | 0.75 –1.0 g i.m. | |
| | (see text) | |

## Fully supervised intermittent regimens

When administration of chemotherapy is advisable on a fully supervised basis the following intermittent regimens are equally effective:

$2HRZ/4H_3R_3$
$2HRZ/4H_2R_2$
$2E_3H_3R_3Z_3/4H_3R_3$
$2S_3H_3R_3Z_3/4H_3R_3$

## Less potent regimens

These must be given for periods longer than 6 months. The following alternatives can be used:

$2SHRZ/6HT$
$2SHRZ/6S_2H_2Z_2$

*Choice of drug regimen.* In technically advanced countries where considerations of cost are only very rarely a factor, the 6-month short course chemotherapy consisting of isoniazid and rifampicin with an initial supplement of two months of pyrazinamide (with or without ethambutol) is widely used. The addition of a fourth drug in the initial phase is valuable in areas where initial drug resistance is prevalent.

In developing countries the choice of regimen is often determined by cost. Short course intensive treatment with rifampicin containing regimens gives a vastly improved rate of cure even if patients default after 2 or 3 months' treatment and if relapse occurs it is almost always with sensitive organisms.

Current evidence suggests that patients with smear negative and culture positive disease may well need a minimum of 6 months' treatment, that patients who are both smear and culture negative require not less than 4 months' treatment and that even 4 months of a 4 drug regimen given 3 times a week may be effective.

Despite these extremely successful modern regimens failure still occurs. The biggest problem is non-compliance with patients who discontinue their treatment too early or become irregular drug takers. Treatment failure is sometimes due to failure on the part of the physicians and others to prescribe regimens sufficiently accurately. It should be standard practice that all patients with tuberculosis should be referred to a clinic experienced and if possible specifically designed to treat this disease.

With regimens that are now widely employed, failure of treatment in patients with initial drug resistance is much less likely to

Table 6.5 Summary of recommended treatment for main opportunistic mycobacterial infections

| Mycobacterial species | Commonest clinical features | Key drugs* |
|---|---|---|
| *kansasii* *szulgai* | Pulmonary disease | Rifampicin and ethambutol +/- isoniazid prothionamide if R or E resistant. **Duration: 9–15 months |
| MAIS complex (see text) | Lymph nodes (pulmonary disease) (Disseminated disease) | Rifampicin, ethambutol and isoniazid. (? + streptomycin ? newer rifampicins in failures). **Duration: 2 years |
| *xenopii* | Pulmonary disease | Rifampicin and ethambutol ? + isoniazid, streptomycin (some strains are sensitive to a number of drugs). **Duration: 2 years |
| *malmoense* | Pulmonary disease | Rifampicin and ethambutol ? + isoniazid. **Duration: 2 years |
| *fortuitum* | Injection abscess Pulmonary disease Post-cardiac surgery | Four drugs from gentamycin, amikacin, streptomycin, erythromycin and prothionamide according to sensitivity tests. **Duration: 15 months |
| *chelonei subspecies abscessus* | Injection abscess Post-cardiac surgery (rarely, mycobacterial dissemination after renal transplantation) | |
| *marinum* | Localised skin granuloma | Rifampicin and ethambutol Duration: until completely cleared |

*Most patients will have had an initial period of treatment with three or four drug regimen.

** In AIDS patients, lifelong.

Taken, with permission, from Horne N W 1990 Modern drug treatment of tuberculosis.

occur. Thus in many technically advanced countries initial drug resistance will be encountered in only one of every two or three hundred patients. The intensive regimens now employed, particularly if both bactericidal drugs rifampicin and pyrazinamide are included, ensure that the number of treatment failures will be negligible.

# DRUGS IN SPECIAL SITUATIONS
## Renal impairment

The level of renal function below which the dose of drug should be reduced depends on whether the drug is entirely eliminated by renal excretion (e.g. streptomycin) and on the seriousness of toxicity e.g. visual impairment due to

---

**Box 6.8   Incidence of mycobacteria causing pulmonary disease**

Common: *kansasii, xenopii, malmoensi* and *Mycobacterium avium intracellulare* complex

Rare: *szulgai, simiae, fortuitum, cheloniae abscessus*

---

**Table 6.6   Arbitrary grading for renal function**

| Grade | GFR (ml/min) | Serum creatinine (approx) $\mu$mol/l |
|---|---|---|
| Mild | 20–50 | 150–300 |
| Moderate | 10–20 | 300–700 |
| Severe | < 10 | > 700 |

---

ethambutol is more important than vomiting due to PAS. A commonly used arbitrary grading for renal function is given in Table 6.6.

Renal function declines with age. The following recommendations are made for treatment in renal impairment or failure:

1. Rifampicin is safest of all as it is excreted entirely in the bile. Isoniazid is relatively safe but if the GFR is less than 10 ml/min the maximum dose used should be 200 mg daily and prophylaxis with pyridoxine given.

2. If the GFR is less than 50 ml/min the dose of streptomycin should be reduced and levels monitored. The same applies to capreomycin. Patients on renal dialysis should be given 0.75 g of streptomycin 4–6 hours before dialysis. If ethambutol must be given, very careful monitoring of serum levels is required although the need to give ethambutol under these circumstances is rare.

## Liver impairment

There is no need to regularly perform liver function tests in patients unless they are alcoholic, elderly or malnourished, or in children under the age of 2 who handle rifampicin less efficiently. The drug should only be discontinued if the liver enzymes continue to rise or if jaundice develops.

## Pregnancy

Isoniazid has not been demonstrated to cause teratogenic effects in animals but the drug does cross the placental barrier. There is as yet no evidence to incriminate isoniazid as a causative

agent in malformations and it is recommended in pregnancy.

Rifampicin has been the subject of debate. The drug has been teratogenic in rodents when given in much greater doses than in routine practice in humans. It is felt therefore that there is no evidence that the current doses of rifampicin used in clinical practice have a teratogenic effect.

There is no evidence that ethambutol or PAS cause congenital malformations. Streptomycin is potentially ototoxic and causes deafness and there are a number of single case reports describing deaf children born to mothers given streptomycin during pregnancy. However even though a causative link has failed to be established with certainty, streptomycin is best avoided in pregnancy if possible. Ethionamide and prothionamide have been shown to be teratogenic and should be avoided. Pyrazinamide, thiacetazone and cycloserine appear safe.

## Tuberculous meningitis

Early diagnosis and treatment vastly improves both survival and freedom from residual neurological defects. The penetration of drugs into the CSF is variable. Streptomycin penetrates only if the meninges are inflamed. Isoniazid penetrates well and remains an essential drug in the management of meningitis. Although initial studies have suggested rifampicin does not penetrate well into the CSF there is evidence that levels of the drug above its MIC for tubercle bacilli are obtained after 6 hours if a dose of 15 mg/kg is administered orally. Pyrazinamide achieves a highly satisfactory CSF level and should be included in all regimens. Ethambutol penetrates well into inflamed meninges in a dose of 25 mg/kg. Theoretically therefore, initial treatment with isoniazid 10 mg/kg, rifampicin 10 mg/kg, pyrazinamide 35 mg/kg with or without ethambutol 15 mg/kg and with or without intrathecal streptomycin for the first 2 to 3 months appears optimal therapy. After the CSF has become normal a continuation phase with rifampicin and isoniazid daily for a total period of 12 months is usually sufficient. The role of corticosteroids in tuberculous meningitis remains debatable and recent studies have shown no benefit from the addition of corticosteroids.

## Tuberculosis in immunosuppressed patients

There is an increasing number of patients now being given immunosuppressive drugs and many of these patients are in an older age group and will have been infected in the past with tuberculosis. Many of them will have abnormal chest X-rays suggestive of scars due to previous infection with tubercle. It is recommended that prior to embarking on long-term suppressive therapy the risk of development of tuberculosis should be carefully assessed in the following manner:

- routine tuberculin testing: if positive give isoniazid prophylaxis, if negative observe
- routine chest and abdominal radiographs. Ifcalcification present give isoniazid prophylaxis. If abnormal give standard antituberculous therapy.

Patients should undergo regular clinical and radiological examination with special reference to the exclusion of tuberculsois. A high index of suspicion is important.

## CHEMOTHERAPY IN EXTRAPULMONARY TUBERCULOSIS

Although most of the studies of short-course tuberculosis therapy have been applied to pulmonary disease, new studies are now emerging to suggest that a similar approach is suitable for extrapulmonary tuberculosis with the exception of tuberculous meningitis.

## Treatment of the primary lesion

There is much evidence to make treating all primary disease worthwhile. This is particularly the case with young children in whom the risk of dissemination, particularly meningitis, is greatest and as dissemination of the infection to the female genital tract is a frequent cause of sterility, treatment of female children with primary tuberculosis assumes additional importance. The need for treatment of children in older age groups is more controversial but prevention of morbidity in later years in the form of skeletal or genito-urinary disease makes treatment a reasonable option. Treatment should be with a standard 6-month regimen whenever possible. However, isoniazid prophylaxis is adequate if a positive tuberculin test without demonstrable disease occurs.

Support for the view that manifestations of the disease should be treated by chemotherapy is provided by the experience with pleural effusion. Tuberculous pleural effusions usually appear within a year of primary infection in children and adolescents. In pre-chemotherapy days 25% of patients with pleural effusion subsequently developed obvious progressive pulmonary tuberculosis usually within 2 years. These complications are abolished if all patients with pleural effusion suspected to be tuberculous are treated with chemotherapy for an appropriate period. Large pleural effusions can cause breathlessness and fibrothorax and these problems can be solved by the administration of corticosteroids along with chemotherapy. Prednisolone should be commenced at 40 mg/day and treatment for 6 weeks is usually adequate.

### Tuberculous pericardial effusions

These respond equally well to conventional antituberculosis therapy but steroids should be given early. Miliary tuberculosis was in the past always almost fatal but with standard chemotherapy recovery is now the rule. The dose of isoniazid in miliary disease is 10–12 mg/kg.

### Tuberculous laryngitis

This is distressing and can occasionally histologically and macroscopically be confused for squamous cell carcinoma of the larynx. The bronchial lesions, however, heal well under the influence of drugs.

*Lymph node tuberculosis* is variable in its response to chemotherapy. Even after prolonged treatment nodes may enlarge, erupt and form abscesses. Early incision of the abscess and evacuation of the pus prevents the occurrence of unsightly scarring. The early introduction of steroids helps reduce the size of large and unsightly lymph nodes.

In primary pulmonary tuberculosis bronchial luminal narrowing can occur due to extrinsic compression from enlarged tuberculous hilar lymph nodes. Late sequelae such as bronchiectasis can be often prevented by the early introduction of corticosteroids to reduce the size of these nodes.

## ATYPICAL MYCOBACTERIAL INFECTIONS

The atypical or opportunist mycobacteria are ubiquitous in the environment occurring in water and soil and in association with birds, pigs and cattle. As a general rule the isolation of the same opportunistic species from two specimens taken a week apart in association with characteristic radiological or clinical appearances would be an indication for chemotherapy. A problem is created by these infections in that they are commonly resistant to several and in some instances to all antituberculosis drugs. Although many such infections respond to treatment all should be regarded as a serious threat to the patient's survival and the best possible chemotherapy should be prescribed and carefully monitored. Particularly serious are infections with strains including *Mycobacterium avium, Mycobacterium intracellulare, Mycobacterium scrofulacum, Mycobacterium xenopii* and *Mycobacterium fortuitum.*

Certain mycobacteria cause pulmonary disease more commonly than others (Box 6.8).

In Europe the commonest agent is *Mycobacterium kansasii* whereas in areas where AIDS is rife Mycobacterium avium intracellulare is the most frequent causative organism. Multiple drug treatment is required usually for long term. Suggested regimens for the main opportunistic mycobacterial infections are shown in Table 6.5.

## MANAGEMENT OF PATIENTS IN WHOM PRIMARY CHEMOTHERAPY HAS FAILED

When primary chemotherapy has failed the cause is likely to be failure of the patient to have been compliant, the development of acquired resistance or because multiple resistance was initially present. Relapse in patients who have not been treated previously and who have been prescribed one of the modern short course regimens is almost always due to default before treatment has been completed. Such patients can be retreated with the primary drug regimen as relapse is likely to be associated with fully sensitive organisms.

If it is believed that resistance has been acquired because of the use of less potent regimens the following principles are important in coming to a decision:

1. An accurate chemotherapy history.
2. The choice of drugs to be used is more propitious if the sensitivity of the patient's organism is known. If the patient is not ill and the disease is limited it may be reasonable to wait until full bacteriological information is available.
3. It should be remembered that cross-resistance between drugs, e.g. capreomycin and viomycin exists and care must be taken not to include a drug in the regimen that is known to have a risk of cross-resistance.

4. The reserve drugs, at least the majority of the more effective ones, have a high incidence of important side-effects and some of them are particularly hazardous.
5. A large number of patients requiring treatment for drug resistant tuberculosis have co-operated poorly in the past with many social medical and personality problems.
6. Reserve drugs are expensive thus presenting an important problem in developing countries.
7. There is good evidence that the use of three or possibly four drugs gives substantially better results than a two drug regimen. There is also evidence that isoniazid may have a beneficial effect although resistance has been demonstrated in vivo and the drug should be a useful addition to the regimen.
8. The addition of a drug one at a time to a regimen must be avoided.

The duration of the regimen, taking into consideration the above points, should be at least three drugs to which the patient's organism is known to be sensitive. Preferably it should contain three drugs which he has never received before. Thereafter a minimum of two drugs should be continued for at least 12 months after sputum smears are negative.

# CHEMOPROPHYLAXIS OF TUBERCULOSIS

Chemoprophylaxis is used either:

- to prevent the establishment of infection, e.g. in a breastfed child or in mass population studies – this is primary or infection prophylaxis; and
- secondary or disease prophylaxis when it is used in individuals who have been demonstrably infected with mycobacterium.

The discovery of a very safe inexpensive oral drug, isoniazid, which is bactericidal for the tubercle bacillus has made chemoprophylaxis readily available. Ideally isoniazid is given on its own but if there is any question of isoniazid resistance then it should be given in conjunction with rifampicin. The recommended duration of prophylaxis is 12 months with a minimum of 6 months. Studies have shown that prophylaxis reduces the incidence of tuberculosis in at risk populations by two-thirds. As mentioned previously the drug can produce liver disease and it should be given with caution to patients above the age of 35.

The indications for prophylaxis can be summarised as follows:

- It has limited use in developing countries but may be important in areas of high prevalence of HIV infection.
- In some geographical situations or for psychological reasons separation of the breastfed child from the mother may be inappropriate. In these circumstances isoniazid chemoprophylaxis should be given to the infant until the mother is non-infectious. Isoniazid resistant BCG may be administered concurrently.
- Close contacts of newly diagnosed patients with a positive skin test (5mm or more to 10 IUPPD or Heaf grade II or greater) and who are under 5 years of age should be given chemoprophylaxis. The risk to children aged between 5 and 15 years is extremely low.
- Patients who are newly infected, i.e. who are known to be tuberculin negative in the recent past and have converted.
- There is an increased risk of developing tuberculosis in some clinical conditions such as requiring corticosteroids, malignant disease, diabetes, etc.
- Immigrants from areas of high prevalence of tuberculosis will develop the disease at a much higher rate than the indigenous population and chemoprophylaxis should be considered in such groups.
- In the USA chemoprophylaxis is often advised for tuberculin positive subjects up to the age of 35 with none of the above risk factors.

- Patients who are recommended to have treatment because of the presence of old stable fibrotic lesions observed on the chest X-ray.

However, these patients should not be given monotherapy and should ideally be treated for 4 months with a minimum of two drugs.

---

FURTHER READING

Horne N W 1990 Modern drug treatment of tuberculosis. Chest Heart and Stroke Association.

Rieder H L 1992 Misbehaviour of a dying epidemic: a call for less spectacular and better surveillance. Tubercle and Lung Disease 73: 181–183.

CHAPTER CONTENTS

**Introduction   115**

**Epidemiology   115**

**Treatment--the problems   117**
Cytotoxic chemotherapy   118
   Cyclophosphamide   118
   Adriamycin   119
   Vinca alkaloids   119
   Etoposide   120
   Cisplatin   120
   Methotrexate   121

**Chemotherapy for small cell lung cancer   121**

**Chemotherapy for non–small cell lung cancer   124**

**Radiotherapy for non–small cell lung cancer   125**

**The paraneoplastic syndromes   127**
   Hypercalcaemia   127
   The syndrome of inappropriate ADH
      secretion   127
   Ectopic ACTH syndrome   128
   Hypertrophic pulmonary osteoarthropathy   128
   Lambert Eaton myasthenic syndrome   128

**Terminal care in lung cancer   128**
   Pain   128
   Cough   129
   Dyspnoea   129
   Pericarditis   129
   Anorexia   129

# 7

# Lung cancer

## INTRODUCTION

Lung cancer remains the commonest cancer in the Western world, and its incidence is rising steadily in third world countries where smoking prevalence is extremely high. The prospects of cure remain bleak. Screening programmes aimed at early detection have failed to usefully influence survival. Surgical resection remains the best chance of cure, but for the great majority of cases palliative treatment is all one can offer. This can be attempted with radiotherapy, chemotherapy, a combination of both or simply with supportive measures and pain relief.

This chapter discusses the drug treatment of lung cancer including the use of cytotoxic chemotherapy in small cell carcinoma of the bronchus.

## EPIDEMIOLOGY

Lung cancer has shown the greatest relative and absolute rise in mortality of any tumour this century in England and Wales. In the USA it has been increasing in incidence at up to 10% per year since the 1930s at least, although during the past decade there has been a levelling off, particularly in males. In the USA approximately 120 000 men die per annum, and the figure for women is 34 000; virtually the same as for breast cancer. Recent incidence rates show that for the first time since 1937 there was a significant fall in lung cancer rates among white American men and also in men in England and Wales.

The incidence of lung cancer in women is still increasing and appears to follow 20 years behind the male pattern. Age-specific mortality data show clear differences. While mortality rates continue to increase among the elderly, death rates for lung cancer among young people are now falling. Furthermore this decline in mortality began first in the youngest age group. Figure 7.1 analyses data for England and Wales relating the year of birth to the death rate in age cohorts of 5 years for men and women. Each vertical set of points represents the mortality rate at different ages for persons born during a 10-year period surrounding the central year of birth. Male mortality at each age reaches a peak in the generation born between 1901 and 1916, but in women, although the pattern is similar, the peak death rate is in those born during the 1920s. Thus, there is a cohort of elderly people in the population with a high incidence of lung cancer, and the average age of sufferers will therefore rise at least for the next few years.

The single most important factor in the causation of lung cancer is cigarette consumption.

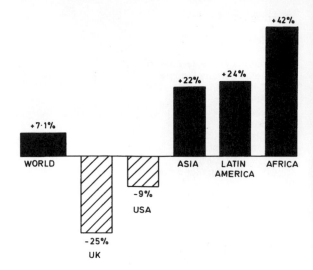

**Fig. 7.2** The changing incidence of tobacco consumption worldwide.

The association was first noticed by Doll and Peto in 1953 in a survey of male English GPs. Whilst great efforts have been made to reduce smoking habits in the Western world with no

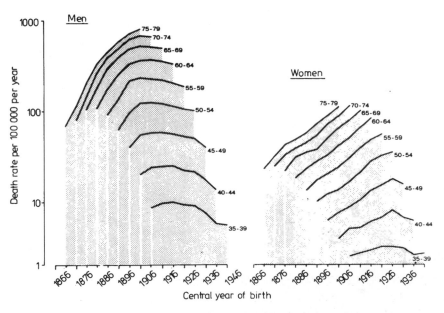

**Fig. 7.1** Age specific mortality from lung cancer in England and Wales during 1941–1980 plotted against central year of birth (From Coggan & Acheson 1983; Thorax 38: 721–723, with permission).

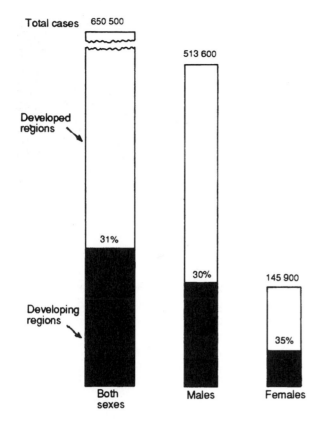

Total cases    650 500

Developed
regions

31%

Developing
regions

Both
sexes

513 600

30%

Males

145 900

35%

Females

**Fig. 7.3**   The incidence of lung cancer in developed and developing countries.

Box 7.1    Lung cancer: cell types and doubling times

| Cell type | % | Doubling time (days) |
|---|---|---|
| Small cell | 20 | 30 |
| Squamous | 50 | 60–90 |
| Adeno | 25 | 90–150 |
| Large (undifferentiated) | 15 | 60–150 |

little success (Fig. 7.2), there has been an alarming rise in Asia, Latin America and Africa. For example, the incidence of smoking in men is above 70% in most of South East Asia and above 50% in most Latin American countries. The incidence for women is still much lower, e.g. 2% in Malaysia where 56% of men smoke. However, although the incidence of lung cancers in developing regions is around 30% (Fig. 7.3), it is rising fast and is already present in a higher percentage of women than men.

## TREATMENT – THE PROBLEMS

In non-small cell lung cancer (NSCLC: squamous, adeno and large cell tumour types), surgery remains the only treatment that offers a possible chance of cure (i.e. 5-year disease-free survival). However, only 15–20% of patients with newly diagnosed NSCLCs go to surgery and of these only a third to a quarter are likely to be alive and disease-free at 5 years. The rest will relapse, either within the chest or at an extrathoracic site. These, and the huge majority of patients with non-small cell lung cancer who were never considered candidates for resection are destined to die from uncontrollable disease.

All these patients will at some stage be given drug therapy for one reason or another during the final stages of their lives. For the great majority this will be to improve or control symptoms such as anorexia, nausea, pain or non-metastatic manifestations of the disease. Some will receive radiotherapy for palliative purposes and a minority may be given cytotoxic chemotherapy.

Whilst NSCLCs comprise 80% of all lung cancers, the role of cytotoxic drug therapy is much more prominent in the remaining cell type: small cell lung cancer (SCLC) (Box 7.1). Small cell cancers have the fastest growth rates of the four main cell types and this rapid growth potential means that at presentation the disease is often very bulky with extensive mediastinal nodal involvement obvious on the chest radiograph, together with clinical evidence of extrathoracic spread. Hence this cell type is virtually never resectable. It has a much greater responsiveness to cytotoxic chemotherapy than non-small cell lung cancers and this has become the mainstay of therapy. However, as will be discussed, relapse is almost inevitable and the subsequent management becomes symptom-related and purely palliative.

**Table 7.1   Objective average response to single agent chemotherapy in lung cancer**

| Drug | Small cell* | Squamous** | Adeno** | Large** |
|------|-------------|------------|---------|---------|
| Ifosfamide | 63 | 27*** | 23*** | 36*** |
| Vincristine | 42 | 10 | 20 | 0 |
| Epipodophyllotoxin | 40 | 25 | 12 | 0 |
| Cyclophosphamide | 33 | 20 | 20 | 23 |
| Methotrexate | 30 | 25 | 30 | 12 |
| Adriamycin | 30 | 20 | 15 | 25 |
| CCNU | 15 | 30 | 20 | 17 |
| Cis Platinum | 35 | 20 | 12 | 13 |

| *   | Hansen & Rorth (1979, 1980) |
| **  | Souhami (1984) |
| *** | Constanzi et al (1982); Harrison et al (1982) |

## Cytotoxic chemotherapy

Lung cancers, in particular SCLC, show a high rate of response (i.e. an at least 50% reduction in tumour volume in 2 perpendicular diameters) to several drugs when given as single agents (Table 7.1). The recent introduction of newer agents (Table 7.2) has provoked much interest, but although several of these drugs are very active, particularly in SCLC, they have had little impact on survival. Individual drugs are discussed briefly below.

### Cyclophosphamide

This is an alkylating agent of the nitrogen mustard type. It is widely used as an immunosuppressive drug in pulmonary medicine (e.g. in Wegener's granulomatosis, fibrosing alveolitis, other eosinophilic vasculitides) and not just in lung cancer. It is one of the most active agents against SCLC.

Its mode of action is complex. Cyclophosphamide is inactive and metabolised in the liver to an active metabolite – phosphoramide mustard – which alkylates or binds with many biologically important proteins including DNA and RNA, so that the genetic processes of both replication and transcription are impeded.

Mode of administration: cyclophosphamide can be given orally or intravenously. Oral dosage is unusual for lung cancer but is commonly advocated for chronic conditions such as cryptogenic fibrosing alveolitis and Wegener's granulomatosis. The standard intravenous dose is 800–1000 mg/m$^2$ given as a slow bolus injection.

In common with other cytotoxic agents, cyclophosphamide may produce many side-effects. Nausea and vomiting occur and are treated symptomatically. Myelosuppression is unavoidable and is the dose-limiting factor. The white cell count nadir occurs 7 to 10 days after an i.v. bolus dose and full recovery takes another 10 to 14 days, limiting cycle frequency to approximately every 3 weeks. Alopecia is inevitable following conventional cytotoxic doses, and takes 3 to 6 weeks to develop. Regrowth occurs after stopping therapy. Cystitis may occur with high

**Table 7.2   Phase II responses in new single agents in small cell lung cancer**

| Drug | No. of pts. | Average responding (%) |
|------|-------------|------------------------|
| Vindesine | 74 | 19 |
| Teniposide | 36 | 19 |
| Mitoxantrone | 6 | 53 |
| Streptozotocin | 41 | 0 |
| Vinblastine | 34 | 0 |

dose therapy (greater than 3 $g/m^2$) and is due to the metabolite acrolein which is toxic to the epithelium of the urinary tract. Haemorrhagic cystitis can occur, particularly with high dose therapy and can be fatal if the drug is not discontinued. The cystitis can be prevented by giving 2-mecaptoethane sulphonate (MESNA) intravenously during and for 12 hours post cyclosphosphamide. MESNA reacts specifically with acrolein and blocks the toxic reaction. Additional hydration, even with MESNA, and always with conventional doses of cyclophosphamide will also minimise the risk of chemical cystitis.

Pulmonary fibrosis is documented as a complication of cyclophosphamide. However, although this is rarely a problem in patients with lung cancer as the duration of administration of cyclophosphamide is relatively short, the development of symptoms can begin within 2 weeks. Cyclophosphamide may also cause a hypersensitivity reaction with urticaria, angiooedema and bronchospasm, but the incidence is very low. The more typical reaction is one of exertional dyspnoea secondary to pulmonary inflammation and oedema. Late inspiratory crackles, fever and pleuritic chest pain can develop. The radiological picture is non-specific and typical of many conditions associated with bilateral basal shadowing or profuse pulmonary oedema. The reaction usually responds to steroids, but progression to death has been reported.

Cyclophosphamide, especially in high doses, seems to sensitise the lung to radiation pneumonitis following conventional doses of radiotherapy. Intense pneumonitis usually with parenchymal destruction, cough and severe dyspnoea has been reported in patients given high dose cyclophosphamide (200 mg/kg) followed by radiotherapy for small cell lung cancer.

Interestingly, pre-dosing with small quantities of cyclophosphamide (50 mg/kg) about 1 to 2 weeks prior to conventional doses seems to protect the lungs of experimental animals from cyclophosphamide-induced pulmonary damage and there is also evidence that this confers some protection to the bone marrow.

### Adriamycin

Adriamycin (or doxorubicin) is a cytotoxic anthracene antibiotic. Its mode of action is not certain, but seems to involve its concentration in cell nuclei where it binds to and disrupts the structure of DNA. It also forms 'free radicals' and may have direct effects on the integrity of lipid membranes, those actions possibly explaining its toxic and dose-limiting effect on normal cells.

Adriamycin is given intravenously as an infusion over about 1 hour. The standard dose is 50 $mg/m^2$. It is rapidly metabolised by the liver to the active substance adriamycinol. Over 70% of its secretion is biliary and 10% renal although the urine can remain red for up to 48 hours after administration.

Its major side-effect is bone marrow suppression, the white cell count reaching its nadir after 10 to 14 days and taking up to 3 weeks following the dose to recover. It is also toxic to the heart muscle and in cancer chemotherapy the dose limit is usually 400 $mg/m^2$ to prevent either serious arrhythmias or a cardiomyopathy.

Irradiation of the chest, especially the mediastinum, if followed by further administration of adriamycin, can cause an intense pneumonitis within the irradiated field. This can also have synergistic toxic effects on the heart, especially if alkylating agents (cyclophosphamide, ifosfamide, chlorambucil or CCNU) are used concurrently.

Tissue necrosis can occur with other cytotoxic agents such as cyclophosphamide and is especially severe if adriamycin finds its way into extravascular tissues. Other side-effects include buccal ulceration, vomiting, diarrhoea and alopecia.

### Vinca alkaloids

There are three vinca alkaloids; vincristine, vinblastine and vindesine, and of these vincristine appears the most active in lung cancer. All three are derived from the periwinkle plant and are similar in properties and structure. They differ mainly in side-effects – the main one with vincristine being peripheral neuropathy, and with vinblastine myelosuppression. Vindesine may cause both. The peripheral neuropathy is due to demyelination and axonal degeneration. It is dose-dependent and is commoner and occurs earlier in elderly patients. The early symptoms include paraesthesiae of the finger tips with associated sensory loss. The ankle jerk is also lost early. Treatment should be reduced by 50% at this stage and symptoms may remain, but not worsen. If they worsen the drug must be stopped. Further administration can lead to wrist and foot drop which are very slow to recover. Autoimmune neuropathy can also occur early causing constipation, intestinal ileus and urinary retention. Other rare side-effects include cardiotoxicity, lung fibrosis and inappropriate ADH secretion.

The vinca alkaloids are all administered intravenously. The standard dose of vincristine is 1.4 mg/m$^2$, but the total dose should not exceed 2 mg. Vindesine is given at a dose of up to 5 mg/m$^2$. The drug can be given as a slow intravenous bolus. It is not myelosuppressive and therefore can be given relatively frequently. Neurotoxicity has to be carefully watched for and the dose halved at the onset of any symptoms.

## Etoposide

Etoposide is a semi-synthetic derivative of podophyllotoxin which is an active component of the naturally occurring substance podophyllin, an established medication for treating warts which comes from the root of the mandrake plant. The intracellular mode of action of etoposide is not known, but it seems to inhibit DNA synthesis at the pre-mitotic stage of cell division.

Although myelotoxic, etoposide can be given over several days as part of a course of chemotherapy. The usual intravenous dose is 100–200 mg/m$^2$ on days 1–3, depending on whether other myelosuppressant drugs are also given. It is administered in 250–500 ml of normal saline over 30–60 minutes.

Etoposide is available as an oral preparation, but absorption is variable both within the same individual and between individuals. The total oral dose is usually twice the intravenous dose e.g. 100 mg orally 8 hourly for 9 doses. However other schedules including 50 mg/day for 14 or 21 days have been shown to be very active in small cell lung cancer. Unexpected marrow toxicity can occur, presumably dependent on more efficient uptake than predicted.

Etoposide is unpalatable and is no longer provided as drinking ampoules but as large 50 and 100 mg capsules. The therapeutic efficacy is more predictable when given intravenously but nevertheless oral etoposide has a useful role in lung cancer chemotherapy. Alopecia develops, but nausea is less common than with the alkylating agents.

The metabolism of etoposide is hepatic and it is renally excreted both in unchanged and metabolised forms. Conventionally, oral and intravenous doses are given over 1 to 3 days every 21 days to allow recovery of myelosuppression, but low dose daily etoposide in 10-day courses is well-tolerated, effective and safe.

## Cisplatin

Cisplatin and carboplatin are both platinum analogues thought to cause their cytotoxic effect by forming cross-linkages in and between DNA strands. Carboplatin is as effective a drug as cisplatin and is less nephrotoxic and causes less vomiting, but is prohibitively expensive and hardly used. Cisplatin is very nephrotoxic and can cause renal tubular necrosis. The intensity of nausea and vomiting associated with cisplatin has become much more controllable with antiemetic regimes including dexamethasone and high dose, or infused, metoclopramide. Alternatively, the 5 HT3 receptor antagonist antiemetics, together with dexamethasone, are highly effective. Myelotoxicity from cisplatin is predictable and similar to other agents. Neuro-toxicity usually occurs as a sensory peripheral neuropathy and occasionally causes tinnitus.

Cisplatin is given intravenously and non-ezymatic conversion to inactive metabolites occurs and the platinum becomes heavily tis-sue-bound. Excretion is renal and the drug should be avoided if the serum creatinine is elevated and a 24-hour clearance is 25% below the normal range. Careful hydration is essential in all patients receiving the drug.

The dose of cisplatin depends on whether other myelosuppressive drugs are being given concomitantly. It is generally given in smaller doses in this predominantly elderly population compared to patients with lymphoma, etc. because of the risk of nephrotoxicity. Vomiting is also a problem and hydration has to be thorough, causing a potential problem of fluid overload in elderly patients. The usual dose in lung cancer chemotherapy is 30–60 mg/m$^2$ given intravenously in 250 ml of normal saline over 1 hour. This is usually preceded by a litre of intravenous fluid and followed by at least a further litre with a diuretic if the urine output is unsatisfactory.

### Methotrexate

This is an antimetabolite which competitively inhibits the enzyme dihydrofolate reductase, thereby preventing the formation of reduced folate which is required for purine and pyrami-dine synthesis.

Methotrexate is available as both oral and intravenous preparations. Although some low dose chemotherapy regimens include oral methotrexate, particularly in the elderly, most patients receive the drug intravenously. The dose again varies dependent on concomitant medication, but most regimens administer 30–50 mg/m$^2$ as a slow intravenous bolus.

The important side-effects are myelotoxicity, especially the white cells and mucosal inflam-mation and ulceration. Buccal ulcers can be very painful and troublesome. Gastrointestinal tract ulceration can cause severe diarrhoea. Folinic acid given intravenously will antagonise the

---

**Box 7.2   Major side-effects of cytotoxic agents**

| Myelotoxicity: | Pulmonary fibrosis: |
|---|---|
| Cyclophosphamide | Cyclophosphamide |
| Ifosfamide | Methotrexate |
| Cisplatin | Adriamycin |
| Etoposide | Bleomycin* |
| Methotrexate | CCNU |
| Adriamycin | |

\* Not given for lung cancer

---

effects of methotrexate. Particular care has to be taken if pleural or peritoneal fluid is present when methotrexate is administered. This causes methotrexate to be stored in the fluid compart-ments, prolonging its excretion and causing both excessive marrow suppression and buccal ulceration. All cases with such 'third space' fluid should be given folinic acid 6 hourly for 24 hours starting 24 hours post the methotrexate dose. Major side-effects of drugs are listed in Box 7.2.

## CHEMOTHERAPY FOR SMALL CELL LUNG CANCER

Chemotherapy for small cell lung cancer was associated with considerable optimism in the mid 1970s when an increased median survival was achieved by using combination chemo-therapy with three to four drugs cycled every 3 weeks. Radiation therapy to the primary tumour site and mediastinum was commonly added before or between chemotherapy cycles in an attempt to improve tumour control at the primary site. A decade later, however, it is proving difficult to extend the duration of sur-vival further with the medication currently available.

In studies in unselected patients, those pre-senting with limited disease (i.e. confined to one hemithorax and the ipsilateral supraclavicular fossa) have a complete response rate to chemotherapy of 30–50% with a median sur-vival of 10 to 16 months. Patients presenting with extensive disease (i.e. including at least one extrathoracic site) have a 15–20% complete response rate with median survival of 6 to 12 months. Although early studies on selected patients suggested that a significant proportion might be cured, analyses of patients alive at 2 years from diagnosis and treatment are less sanguine. A study of 1580 cases of small cell lung cancer in general hospital practice in Seattle found only 2.4% alive at 5 years. Of 874 patients treated at the Finsen Institute in Copenhagen, only 7.6% were alive at 18 months. Furthermore the risk of relapse from small cell lung cancer in this group of patients reached 46% by 5 years after the end of treatment and the risk of dying from a second cancer (usually a non-small cell lung cancer) rose to 32% at 5 years. However, 38 of 54 disease-free survivors were able to resume their pre-diagnosis life style and occupation. In Britain the 2-year survival in an analysis of 3681 patients entered into clinical trials was 8.5% for those presenting with limited disease and 2.2% for extensive disease.

Attempts to improve both the median and long-term survival for patients with small cell lung cancer have included a variety of strategies. 'Maintenance' chemotherapy has been given where, after the initial induction period with cyclical chemotherapy, the same or different drugs are continued at either lower doses or at longer intervals in an attempt to prolong the duration of remission. Doses have also been increased beyond conventional levels in some studies, sometimes using autologous bone marrow transplantation to shorten the period of aplasia. This has been done either as initial induction therapy or as 'late intensification' to consolidate or prolong remission. The use of cyclical alternating combinations of drugs considered to be non-cross resistant has been assessed and there has been continued exploration of new drugs and new drug combinations in intensive regimens.

None of these approaches have yet made a major impact. The newer agents such as etoposide, teniposide, ifosfamide, cisplatin and carboplatin have been shown to be highly active as single agents or in combination (e.g. etoposide and cisplatin). These drugs are used in many chemotherapy regimens, but no consistent improvement in median or long-term survival has yet been found in unselected cases. Typical combinations of chemotherapy are summarised in Table 7.3.

Trials assessing the impact on survival of the addition of radiotherapy to chemotherapy have shown no major advantage. Whilst it is acknowledged that radiotherapy to the primary tumour site and mediastinum decreases the local relapse rate at this site, patients die

**Table 7.3    Commonly used cytotoxic regimens in small cell lung cancer**

| Regimen A | *every 21 days* |
|---|---|
| i) Cisplatin | $50 \text{ mg/m}^2$ |
| Etoposide | $120 \text{ mg/m}^2$ days 1, 2, 3 |
| alternating with | |
| ii) Cyclophosphamide | $600 \text{ mg/m}^2$ |
| Adriamycin | $50 \text{ mg/m}^2$ |
| Vincristine | 2 mg |
| **Regimen B** | *every 21 days* |
| Cyclophosphamide | $1 \text{ g/m}^2$ |
| Doxorubicin | $40 \text{ mg/m}^2$ |
| Vincristine | $1 \text{ mg/m}^2$ (max 2 mg) |
| **Regimen C** | *every 21 days* |
| Cyclophosphamide | $1 \text{ g/m}^2$ |
| Vincristine | $1.4 \text{ mg/m}^2$ (max 2 mg) |
| Etoposide | $80 \text{ mg/m}^2$ on days 1, 2, 3 |
| **Regimen D** | *every 28 days* |
| Carboplatin | $300 \text{ mg/m}^2$ |
| Etoposide | $100 \text{ mg/m}^2$ i.v. days 1, 2, 3 |
| **Regimen E** | *every 21 days* |
| Etoposide | $120 \text{ mg/m}^2$ days 1, 2, 3 |
| Cyclophosphamide | $1 \text{ g/m}^2$ |
| Methotrexate | $35 \text{ mg/}^2$ |
| Vincristine | $1.3 \text{ mg/}^2$ (max 2 mg) |

primarily because of the failure of chemotherapy to destroy metastatic deposits.

A recent meta analysis of all studies randomising newly diagnosed patients to chemotherapy alone versus chemotherapy plus radiotherapy to the primary site has shown a survival advantage of 5% for the combined modality arms. This advantage is maintained out to and beyond 5 years post therapy. Those studies incorporated radiotherapy administered at the beginning of the course of chemotherapy, in the middle or after completion. However whilst it is clear that radiotherapy does conform a survival advantage to patients with small cell lung cancer, it is not clear whether the timing is critical. This is the subject of several current studies.

With this background of lack of progress, some recent studies have assessed on the optimal duration of administration of chemotherapy. There is no doubt that the majority of patients respond to chemotherapy with considerable improvement in their presenting symptoms and in parameters that attempt to measure quality of life. Most patients, especially the majority who have extensive disease, obtain only short remissions before disease progression and death. The balance between effective therapy and minimal toxicity is therefore crucial.

Several studies have addressed the question of the value of maintenance chemotherapy following the initial response, and also the length of initial chemotherapy with or without further chemotherapy on relapse. In 1984 Feld published two sequential non-randomised studies. The first comprised 147 patients treated by three courses of cyclophosphamide, adriamycin and vincristine (CAV) with thoracic irradiation followed by a year of maintenance chemotherapy with CCNU, procarbazine and methotrexate. Their second study was of 320 patients (153 limited disease and 167 extensive disease) treated by six courses of CAV and thoracic irradiation, but no maintenance chemotherapy. In the latter study the median survival for patients with limited and extensive disease was 49 and 34 weeks respectively and similar to those in the initial study which included 1 year of maintenance chemotherapy.

Three large randomised studies of chemotherapy duration have recently been published. One randomised 616 patients to receive either four or eight courses of chemotherapy and, at relapse, to receive either symptomatic treatment or relapse chemotherapy with different agents to those used during initial chemotherapy. The study showed that patients allocated to receive four courses of initial chemotherapy only (with no further therapy at relapse) had a median survival of 30 weeks, which was significantly inferior to the other three treatment arms (median survivals of 39–42 weeks). This difference was more marked for the responding populations.

In an MRC study 497 patients were given six cycles of a four-drug regimen with additional radiotherapy between courses two and three to patients with limited disease who responded. At the completion of the initial six cycles, patients whose disease remained controlled were randomised to either no further chemotherapy or six further courses of the same drugs but at slightly longer intervals (4 weeks instead of 3 weeks). The median survival of all patients entered was 39 weeks with no overall advantage for patients who received the maintenance therapy.

The French small cell lung cancer group randomised 106 patients with complete response after six courses of chemotherapy to a further six courses, or to no more chemotherapy, which again confirmed no survival advantage.

There still are few studies which address the question of quality of life during and after chemotherapy. A recent study evaluated eight parameters aimed at assessing quality of life and compared them in patients receiving four and eight cycles during the second part of the treatment when they were receiving courses five to eight or no further therapy. All the quality of life measures deteriorated during courses five to eight, particularly as therapy progressed. This reflects the disadvantage of the second four courses of chemotherapy, but must be offset against the longer median survival associated with eight courses of chemotherapy. However, a separate study of the impact of initial chemotherapy also showed a considerable quality of life benefit during treatment, approximately 65% of those with symptoms obtaining relief from pain, cough, shortness of breath, superior vena caval obstruction, or dysphagia.

It is reasonable to conclude that six courses of chemotherapy is a reasonable duration of treatment. Maintainance chemotherapy or further treatment at relapse is not useful. The question still remains whether all patients with SCLC should be treated for this period. For patients with extensive disease this would seem a reasonable decision. For some patients with extensive disease, and several with limited disease, more intensive therapy may be justified from data assessing prognostic factors for survival made at the time of diagnosis. Those patients destined to have the greatest chance of long-term survival are those with a good (high) performance status and normal biochemistry; particularly albumin, sodium, alkaline phosphatase and other liver enzymes at the time of diagnosis. Studies evaluating these parameters can now identify the majority of patients who are likely to be long-term survivors. It remains to be seen whether patients in a good prognostic category can improve their survival with more intensive chemotherapy. If not, these patients should also receive no more than six courses until new and better drugs become available (Box 7.3).

## CHEMOTHERAPY FOR NON-SMALL CELL LUNG CANCER

In spite of more than a decade of intensive research there is no clear indication that cytotoxic chemotherapy should occupy a major place in the management of NSCLC. Although there have been hundreds of studies, little attempt has been made to compare carefully matched patient populations, and trials have usually included small numbers of patients only, usually with no control data. There are only five placebo-controlled studies in the liter-

---

**Box 7.3  Chemotherapy in small cell lung cancer**

1. 6 cycles is optimal
2. No advantage for maintenance therapy
3. No advantage with alternating 'non-cross resistant' drugs
4. No advantage in more intensive chemotherapy
5. Mediastinal irradiation benefits survival
6. Prognostic indicators at diagnosis are the most important discriminators of response

---

ature, most investigators using either historical controls, which have many potential flaws, or comparing the results of one regimen with another. To date, 15 drugs have been studied in more than 100 patients with NSCLC and the overall response rates of the most active agents are summarised in Table 7.1. The three most active drugs appear to be ifosfamide, cisplatin and mitomycin C. Most studies only record response data (i.e. at least a 50% or greater tumour reduction measured in two perpendicular diameters) and there is very little data on the impact of chemotherapy on the quality of life.

The value of combination chemotherapy is also not proven, there being only a small number of prospective randomised studies comparing the response rates achieved to those in single agent studies. Of these, only two show unequivocal evidence of higher response rates for the combination under test and only one study claimed an improved survival time for patients treated with a combination regimen. A recent report of 486 good performance status patients with metastatic NSCLC were given one of the four most active combinations of chemotherapy and showed that the response rates for the regimens ranged between 17–31%, but there was absolutely no impact on median survival of 24.5 weeks. The durations of responses in this study were short (1 to 3 months) and only 12 patients survived more than 2 years. There were 20 treatment related deaths as part of wider significant toxicity. The poorer the performance status of the patients entering the study, the lower were the chances of a response and the higher the risk of toxicity.

A small number of studies have evaluated combination chemotherapy versus best supportive care in patients with advanced NSCLC. None has shown a clinically worthwhile advantage for chemotherapy. Whilst some patients responded well and had a prolonged survival, many of those who did less well suffered toxic side-effects from treatment.

It seems clear therefore that there is no justification for the administration of chemotherapy to patients with NSCLC outside the forum of a controlled clinical trial.

Recently the three most active single agents in NSCLC: ifosfamide, mitomycin C and cisplatin, have been given to patients with inoperable disease as a phase II study. Of 74 patients, 30 (45%) achieved a response and seven (11%) a complete response. The overall response was 56%, with 29 of 43 responses in the 50 patients with limited disease. The median duration of response was 8.75 months and the median survival for the whole group 9.2 months (Cullen et al, 1988). This response rate, considerably greater than for any other combination of chemotherapy for NSCLC, has been confirmed in a similar study by our own group, and is now being assessed in a controlled study of this combination of chemotherapy followed by radiotherapy against radiotherapy alone in inoperable cases of NSCLC where disease is confined to a radiotherapy field.

## RADIOTHERAPY IN NON-SMALL CELL LUNG CANCER

Radiotherapy can potentially be given at several stages during the course of lung cancer:

- preoperatively
- instead of surgery
- post-resection
- to inoperable patients with limited disease in radical dosage and
- to inoperable patients as palliative therapy either to the primary tumour or symptomatic metastases.

*Preoperative radiotherapy.* This has been used in a few uncontrolled studies to sterilise or reduce the bulk of the primary mass, often including the mediastinum. However, the postoperative survival data are no better than those for surgery alone and this approach has been abandoned.

Early studies of superior sulcus tumours suggested that survival was improved by preoperative irradiation when compared to surgery alone. However subsequent studies have also failed to confirm this advantage and have shown equally good results for surgery alone.

*Instead of surgery.* Irradiation of primary tumours that appeared operable but were not resected because of either medical contraindications or patient's refusal, appeared to do just as well with radiotherapy as with surgery in an early study. This 1956 study with carefully selected cases contained only patients with squamous cell cancers and achieved a 5-year survival rate of 22.5%. However, subsequent trials have failed to even approach these results, and more typically a 1-year survival figure of 36% with only 6% of patients alive at 5 years was reported in a later study.

*Post-resection.* The role of post-operative irradiation has for long been confusing. Uncontrolled studies in the 1970s suggested a survival advantage for all non-small cell types for post-resection irradiation, even if the resection appeared curative. However the results from two recent large randomised studies firmly refute this. A European study with 175 patients, all with non-small cell types undergoing curative resection, with no tumour extension beyond the lung and no involvement of lymph nodes, were randomised to either just follow-up or 60 Gy radiotherapy in 6 weeks, beginning 3 to 4 weeks post-operatively. There was no increase in survival in the irradiated group who in fact had a lower 5-year survival (24% versus 43% for the control group), but the difference was not statistically significant. However, irradiation decreased the rate of local relapse with 50% of relapses in the control group and 85% in the radiation group being extrathoracic.

Another study of squamous cell tumours in 1986 with a similar design to that above, included 210 eligible patients. The dose of radiotherapy was 50 Gy given 28 days post-surgery in the active arm of the study. The two groups were well-matched both anthropometrically and for tumour stage. There was no evidence that radiotherapy improved survival, and although the local recurrence rates were somewhat reduced in the radiotherapy arm, the decreases were not significant. In N2 disease (mediastinal node involvement) the recurrence rate was significantly reduced but survival was not because of the high rate of emergence of extrathoracic disease.

Post-operative irradiation to patients known to have had a non-curative resection also achieves no survival advantage. Results show a 5–8% five-year survival rate only.

*Inoperable patients.* Radical radiotherapy is also offered in inoperable patients whose disease appears limited to one hemithorax, with or without involvement of the ipsilateral supraclavicular fossa, but still not very bulky disease. Some investigators refute the claims of the majority that radical radiotherapy confers no definite short-term nor long-term survival advantage to these patients, but most accept the high chance of failure because of occult extrathoracic disease and imperfect control of the local intrathoracic tumour bulk. In most unselected studies, the 5-year survival rate with radical radiotherapy up to 60 Gy is 5%. Earlier randomised studies of radiotherapy versus conservative therapy in the USA and in Oxford which gave 40 to 50 Gy failed to show any advantage for treatment, although these studies have been criticised for including small cell tumours, using older orthovoltage radiation equipment and failing to show that the two groups in each study were perfectly balanced.

Attempts to improve the effectiveness of radiotherapy with hyperbaric oxygen, and various radiosensitizing drugs such as misonidazole and small doses of cisplatin have failed to establish a clear-cut advantage. Currently, the most interesting possibility is superfractionation techniques where intensive treatment is given 3 times a day for 2 to 3 weeks instead of conventional daily dosages.

*Palliative radiotherapy.* The value of radiotherapy in palliating distressing symptoms is beyond dispute and improves the quality of life for these patients. However, the treatment should be carried out at minimum cost in terms of both toxicity and time spent in hospital.

Numerous dose schedules are available, such as 30 Gy in 10 fractions over 2 weeks, 20 Gy in 5 fractions over 5 days, or single fractions of 7.5–10 Gy.

Haemoptysis and cough, the commonest and perhaps most disturbing symptoms, are easily controlled by radiotherapy in up to 80% of sufferers. Dyspnoea caused by bronchial obstruction can be relieved in about half the patients and dysphagia in 80% if it is due to lymph node compression. The syndrome of superior vena caval obstruction is improved in 60% of sufferers, at least in terms of relieving symptoms although the distended neck veins and colaterals may remain visible. Pain due to bone metastases is totally relieved in 50% and partially in a further 30%.

Brain metastases tend to respond relatively poorly to radiotherapy. Initial assessment should be with oral dexamethasone 4 mg q.d.s. for 48 hours which reduces the oedema around the deposit. If acceptable improvement occurs, then radiotherapy can consolidate this and the steroids may be withdrawn. However if the steroid trial makes little difference to the neurological deficit then radiotherapy is unlikely to be additionally effective. Spinal cord compression is relatively common in lung cancer, which accounts for 15% of all cases. Pain or bony tenderness often precedes it and may help to localise the site of compression. Treatment must be prompt, preceded by a myelogram if there is any doubt as to the level of the lesion. Response to radiotherapy is usually incomplete and disappointing. Whilst a decompression laminectomy is the procedure of choice, particularly if the patient has not already been diagnosed to have malignant disease, it is rarely carried out on patients with known lung cancer unless they are in very good general condition and without evidence of other uncontrolled disease. Radiotherapy is excellent palliation in large, painful or unsightly lymphadenopathy.

# THE PARANEOPLASTIC SYNDROMES

These syndromes occur in association with all cell types of lung cancer but are most frequently associated with SCLC. The treatment of some is quite specific and can make a big difference to the welfare of the patient.

## Hypercalcaemia

About 8% of patients with lung cancer develop hypercalcaemia, which is usually associated with the squamous cell type. It is most commonly due to widespread bony metastases causing osteolytic damage, but the primary tumour itself may produce peptide hormones of which parathormone is the commonest. Symptoms of hypercalcaemia include polyuria, dehydration and thirst, constipation, confusion and ultimately renal failure and coma. Treatment depends on the general state of the patient and how advanced the malignant disease is. Palliative therapy alone may be necessary. If, however, the hypercalcaemia is to be treated, the dehydration is initially corrected with i.v. saline 3 to 6 litres per day. The addition of a loop diuretic (e.g. frusemide) is helpful in ensuring a diuresis once rehydration is established. It is common to add intravenous and oral steroids to obtain the benefit of their calcium-lowering properties. Hydrocortisone 100 mg intravenously 6 hourly and, when able to drink, prednisolone 40 mg per day is recommended although the effect of corticosteroids is short. Once the calcium has been lowered it should be determined whether the source (if not yet known) is the primary squamous cell cancer or the presence of bony metastases. If a bone scan is normal or near normal, treatment of the primary tumour can be valuable. Occasionally the tumour is resectable, otherwise radiotherapy can be effective for controlling symptoms. If there are widespread metastases and radiotherapy is not practical, additional therapy is required as hydration and steroids will not hold the metabolic state for more than a few days. Intravenous diphosphonates 30–120 mg are very effective at decreasing calcium levels but are again only successful for a few weeks. However, the dose of diphosphonate can be repeated. Calcitonin subcutaneously or intravenously is also used but is expensive and its effect is not as prolonged as diphosphonate. Mithramycin, a cytotoxic drug, has also a profound calcium-lowering effect given at 25 $\mu$gm/kg as an infusion. It is both renal and myelotoxic and therefore can only be given every 3 weeks or so once marrow suppression has recovered.

## The syndrome of inappropriate antidiuretic hormone secretion (SIADH)

Significant hyponatraemia (sodium < 120 mmol/l) is almost invariably associated with SCLC. It is characterised by dilutional hyponatraemia with a low serum sodium and plasma osmolality (< 260 osmol/kg) and a two- to three-fold increase of urine osmolality. The biochemical abnormalities occur in about 10% of new cases of SCLC and an abnormal response to a water load is found in nearly 50%. Patients may be asymptomatic, but usually complain of anorexia, weakness, nausea, confusion and headaches. If the condition is not corrected coma will ultimately occur.

The corner-stone of therapy used to be water deprivation, but is now demeclocycline 600–1200 mg per day. The drug competes for the ADH renal tubular binding sites and is so effective that no fluid restriction is necessary. The administration of chemotherapy also rapidly corrects the problem in the 90% of patients who respond. Care has to be taken to prevent diabetes insipidus if the response to chemotherapy is good, and care should be taken to discontinue demeclocycline when the electrolytes return to normal in a responding patient.

### Ectopic ACTH syndrome

Although abnormalities in cortisol metabolism are common in SCLC, they rarely cause clinical problems. The natural history of small cell cancer is too short to allow cushingoid symptoms and signs to develop. Hypokalaemia may occur with a metabolic alkalosis with some patients developing progressive pigmentation due to melanophore stimulating hormone (MSH) production.

### Hypertrophic pulmonary osteoarthropathy (HPOA)

Periostitis of the long bones, usually the distal ends of the tibia, fibula, radius and ulnar, causes tenderness, local heat and swelling. Clubbing of the finger ends is present in more than 90% of cases. The pathogenesis of HPOA is obscure, but it is commonest in squamous cell cancer. It also occurs in adenocarcinoma, but is very rare in SCLC. The condition can respond to treatment of the primary tumour if the latter is sufficiently localised. It can also improve occasionally with a vagotomy, but usually requires non-steroidal anti-inflammatory medication for effective control.

### Lambert Eaton myasthenic syndrome (LEMS)

Therapy can specifically improve the management of this rare association with SCLC. It is characterised by progressive proximal muscle weakness, dryness of the mouth and difficulty in swallowing. The onset of symptoms can be remarkably rapid – over a few days. Post-tetanic potentiation can be documented on EMG analysis. Clinically weak muscles get stronger with repeated contraction and absent tendon reflexes return, albeit transiently. The administration of 2,4 amidopyridine 10–20 mg 4–6 times a day can improve muscle strength as may concomitant steroids. However, once again the major control is derived from the tumour mass decreasing on chemotherapy.

## TERMINAL CARE IN LUNG CANCER

The majority of patients with lung cancer are likely to die of the disease within a year of diagnosis. Therefore early introduction of the patient to supportive care is essential. Patients should be aware that skilled help is available to them for advice about symptoms and problems even during any period of therapy intended to alleviate symptoms or even aim at cure. Most respiratory physicians have access to nurse specialists to liaise with their patients as well as a domiciliary nursing team often based within the hospital which specialises in terminal care within the community.

### Pain

Pain is undoubtedly the greatest fear of any patient with lung cancer. Care should be taken to reassure patients that many never suffer pain and, if they do, much can be done. The commonest source of pain is bony disease, which may be easily controllable by simple analgesics such as paracetamol or aspirin. Aspirin is particularly helpful for controlling bone pain, especially when used as an adjunct to opiates in severe cases. Wherever possible analgesics should be given orally. If codeine containing tablets are not adequate then morphine should be introduced earlier rather than later. The development of sustained release morphine preparations (MST, morphine sulphate continuous) has been very valuable. It is available in 10, 30, 60 and 100 mg tablets and is given 12 hourly together with an antiemetic, such as prochlorperazine, if necessary. A gradual increase in dose can provide excellent control for weeks or months. If pain is acute and severe it is advisable to establish control initially with morphine elixir given every 4 hours. Once control has been achieved it is simple to change to MST by merely converting the total daily elixir dose to a b.d. tablet regimen. Localised pain can of course be treated by radiotherapy. Recent studies have convincingly demonstrated that a single fraction of 7–10 Gy is as effective (and much more acceptable for the patient) than a week of smaller daily doses.

### Cough

This can be a most distressing and difficult symptom to treat. Codeine linctus 30–60 mg b.d. or t.d.s. can be effective although, as with all opiates, constipation should be minimised by the early introduction of laxatives such as lactulose, milpar or senna granules. Inhalations of symptomatic remedies such as benzoin eucalyptus and menthol can be helpful. Even nebulised salbutamol is beneficial occasionally. If the cough is dry, a nebulised local anaesthetic such as marcaine 0.3% solution can be useful although the patient should be warned not to attempt to drink whilst their throat is anaesthetised. Ultimately morphine may have to be used to control persistent cough, especially if it is preventing sleep. However, methadone linctus 2–4 mg can also be used with good effect.

### Dyspnoea

There are several causes of breathlessness in lung cancer sufferers. Obstruction of a large central airway can cause severe symptoms which can be relieved either by radiotherapy or laser treatment. Pleural effusions may cause dyspnoea. Once drained, if the lung re-expands a pleurodesis can be attempted with either tetracycline 3 g in 50 ml of normal saline and also 10 ml of 1% lignocaine; bleomycin 90 mg in 50 ml of normal saline, or *Corynebacterium parvum* 7.5 mg in 50 ml of normal saline. All of these work with a 60% success rate provided the instillation is spread around the chest by rotating the patient through 90 degrees every 10 minutes or so for one complete rotation. In the case of *Corynebacterium parvum* the intercostal drain can be removed following the instillation, but for the other agents 2 days of negative intrapleural pressure applied via the intercostal tube is recommended. Should the lung not re-expand following aspiration of fluid there is no purpose in attempting a chemical pleurodesis. Either a surgical pleurectomy should be attempted via a formal thoracotomy or a shunt inserted into the pleural cavity to drain into the periteoneum. Lymphangitis can be a progressive cause of breathlessness which is impossible to relieve. Radiotherapy to the draining hilar lymph nodes is not usually effective. Symptomatic treatment with opiates is the best that can be offered to minimise distress.

Terminal dyspnoea and failure to expectorate secretions can be very distressing, perhaps more to the attending relatives than to the patient. Attempts to dry the secretions with atropine 0.6 mg intramuscularly or hyosine hydrobromide 400–600 $\mu$g 4–6 hourly may be helpful.

### Pericarditis

Direct involvement of the pericardium by lung tumour can cause an effusion and occasionally tamponade. This can be relieved by pericardiocentesis and should it recur, either by surgical exploration of the pericardium to form a window to drain into the peritoneum, or by instilling a sclerosant such as bleomycin 30–45 mg.

### Anorexia

This can be a distressing problem both to the patient and his attenders. The mechanism for the cachexia so common in lung cancer is obscure, but is not helped by the nausea and constipation associated with opiates, buccal ulceration or soreness due to dehydration. Steroids (prednisolone 15–20 mg daily) can be most valuable, but usually help only for a few weeks. Dysphagia can be a superadded problem if mediastinal nodes compress the oesophagus. Radiotherapy often relieves the major symptoms allowing the patient to cope with fluids or semi-solids.

## FURTHER READING

Cullen M H, Jashi R, Chetiyawardana A D, Woodroffe C M 1988 Mitomycin, isosamide and cisplatin in non-small cell lung cancer: treatment good enough to compare. British Journal of Cancer 58: 359–361

Geddes D M, Dones L, Hill E, Law K, Harper P G, Spiro S G, Tobias J S, Souhami R L 1990 Quality of life during chemotherapy for small cell lung cancer: assessment and use of a daily diary card in a randomised trial. European Journal of Cancer 26: 484–492

Souhami R L, Law K 1990 Longevity in small cell lung cancer. British Journal of Cancer 61: 584–589

Spiro S G (ed) 1985 Small cell lung cancer. In: Clinics in Oncology 4, No. 1. W.B. Saunders, London

CHAPTER CONTENTS

**Introduction   131**

**Pulmonary hypertension   131**
Classification and epidemiology     132
Diagnosis   133
  Clinical findings   133
  Investigations   133
Therapeutics   134
  Primary pulmonary hypertension   134
  Secondary pulmonary hypertension   137
Prognosis   139
Therapeutic prospects in pulmonary hypertension   139

**Thromboembolic disease   139**
Epidemiology and definition   139
Deep venous thrombosis   140
  Diagnosis   140
  Prevention and therapy   140
Pulmonary embolus   141
  Acute minor   142
  Acute massive   142
  Chronic thromboembolic disease   142
  Therapy in pulmonary embolus   142
  Management summary: pulmonary embolus   144

**Adult respiratory distress syndrome   145**
New approaches to ventilatory support   145
New modes of ventilation   146
Extracorporeal respiratory support   147
Pharmacological intervention in ARDS   147
New approaches to pharmacotherapy   148
  Steroids   148
  Neutralisation of the effects of endotoxin   149
  Modulation of the cytokine response   149
  Non-steroidal anti-inflammatory drugs   150
  Prostaglandin   150
  Antioxidants   150
  Neutrophil–endothelial cell interaction   150
  Surfactant   151
  Manipulation of the L-arginine pathway   151
Management summary: ARDS   151

# 8

# Pulmonary vascular disease

## INTRODUCTION

Pulmonary vascular disease can involve either the major vessels or the pulmonary capillary bed and may occur as a consequence of conditions affecting the lung parenchyma, the vessels themselves, or a disease process at a distant site. In all cases, the end result is vascular remodelling, occlusion of the vessel lumen, or endothelial injury and disruption. These abnormalities are manifest clinically as pulmonary hypertension (primary or secondary) or alveolar oedema.

## PULMONARY HYPERTENSION

The pulmonary circulation is a low compliance system in which the vascular resistance (PVR) is only 10% of that measured in the systemic circulation (SVR). This difference is largely attributable to the presence of muscular arterioles in systemic vessels that regulate blood flow to the various organs. Although normally PVR is low (< 2.5 mm Hg.L.min) it has the facility to become even smaller as the pressure within it rises. This is due to the recruitment of capillaries that are normally closed or empty, and the distension or increase in calibre of the individual capillary segments. The resistance of any system of blood vessels can be described as follows (Box 8.1):

$$\frac{\text{Input pressure} - \text{Output pressure}}{\text{Blood flow}}$$

---

**Box 8.1    Pulmonary vascular resistance**

The resistance of any system of blood vessels can be described as follows:

Input pressure – Output pressure
_____
            Blood flow

Input pressure is represented by mean pulmonary artery pressure (normally approximately 15 mmHg) and output pressure by left atrial pressure or pulmonary artery occlusion pressure (PAOP). Blood flow is represented by cardiac output. Normal values for these parameters are:

|  | mmHg | Range |
|---|---|---|
| **Pulmonary artery pressure** |  |  |
| Systolic | 25 | 15–30 |
| Diastolic | 9 | 5–12 |
| Mean | 15 | 9–16 |
| Pulmonary artery occlusion pressure (PAOP) | 9 | 5–13 |

---

Input pressure is represented by mean pulmonary artery pressure (normally approximately 15 mmHg) and output pressure by left atrial pressure or pulmonary artery occlusion pressure (PAOP). Blood flow is represented by cardiac output (for normal values see Box 8.1).

## Classification and epidemiology

It is clear that pulmonary vascular resistance may be elevated by a change in any of these parameters. Pulmonary hypertension will therefore accompany any pathological process leading to decreased distensibility of the vessel, or destruction/obstruction of capillaries preventing recruitment. Primary or unexplained pulmonary hypertension is rare and is defined as a mean pulmonary artery pressure above 25 mmHg at rest or above 30 mmHg on exercise in the presence of a cardiac output below 5 l/minute (Box 8.2). The more common secondary pulmonary hypertension is defined similarly but is found in the presence of pulmonary or cardiac disease (Table 8.1, Box 8.3).

The true incidence of primary pulmonary hypertension is unknown. It is a disease principally affecting young adults and women more than men, although a rare familial form is described. The syndrome is associated with a poor prognosis; less than one third of patients are alive within 5 years of diagnosis. The incidence of secondary pulmonary hypertension is even less clear, but is most commonly associated with chronic respiratory failure secondary to chronic obstructive pulmonary disease (COPD). Trends in mortality are difficult to assess, because of changes in disease classification, but mortality is probably falling slightly amongst

---

**Table 8.1    World Health Organisation classification of pulmonary hypertension**

Pulmonary hypertension:

Secondary
Unexplained (primary)
    Plexogenic
    Thromboembolic
    Veno-occlusive

---

**Box 8.2    Criteria for diagnosis of primary pulmonary hypertension**

Mean pulmonary artery pressure above 25 mmHg at rest
                        or
above 30 mmHg on exercise in the presence of a cardiac output below 5 l/minute.

Box 8.3  Conditions leading to secondary pulmonary hypertension

Primary pulmonary hypertension
Secondary pulmonary hypertension
    Chronic thromboembolic disease
    COPD
    Thoracic deformity, kyphoscoliosis
    Fibrotic lung disease

Table 8.2  Clinical findings in pulmonary hypertension

| Symptoms | Signs |
| --- | --- |
| Dyspnoea | Low volume pulse |
| Fatigue | Peripheral cyanosis |
| Syncope | Prominent 'a' or 's' wave in JVP |
| Chest pain | Right ventricular heave |
| Palpitations | Loud P2 |
| Ankle oedema | Third/fourth heart sounds Tricuspid regurgitation Pulmonary regurgitation |

men and rising amongst women. The future depends largely upon the continued prevalence of cigarette smoking. This leads eventually to cor pulmonale, a condition defined as right ventricular hypertrophy associated with pulmonary hypertension occurring secondary to diseases of the lung (see also Ch. 7).

## Diagnosis

Pulmonary hypertension is diagnosed by the demonstration of an elevated PVR in either the absence (primary) or presence (secondary) of cardiopulmonary disease.

### Clinical findings

At presentation dyspnoea, fatigue and syncope or near syncope are the commonest complaints. Raynaud's phenomenon occurs in about 10% of patients, almost all of whom are female. Other symptoms include chest pain, ankle oedema and palpitations. On physical examination, the pulse is of low volume leading to cold extremities and peripheral cyanosis. A right ventricular heave is usually present and auscultation reveals a loud pulmonary component to the second heart sound and often right-sided third and/or fourth sounds. In a proportion of patients, the murmurs of tricuspid and, less commonly, pulmonary incompetence may be heard (Table 8.2). The clinical findings in secondary pulmonary hypertension are identical, but are accompanied by evidence of underlying cardiopulmonary pathology.

### Investigations

All investigations are aimed at excluding cardiopulmonary pathology that might explain any elevation in PVR (Table 8.3).

*Chest radiography.* In secondary pulmonary hypertension there is usually evidence of the cardiopulmonary pathology responsible for the elevation in PVR. Although in a minority of patients with PPH the chest radiograph is normal, more commonly it shows the constellation of changes associated with raised pulmonary

Table 8.3  Practical assessment and management in primary pulmonary hypertension

Chest radiograph
Electrocardiograph
Pulmonary function tests
Arterial blood gases
(Autoantibodies)
Echocardiography
Radioisotope perfusion lung scan
Right heart catheter
Pulmonary angiography
(Open-lung biopsy)

artery pressure: prominence of the pulmonary conus, enlarged hilar vessels and peripheral vascular 'pruning'.

*Haematology.* Up to a third of patients with primary pulmonary hypertension have a positive test for antinuclear antibodies, the significance of which is unclear. Further investigation is directed principally at excluding other causes for the pulmonary hypertension and documenting its severity.

*Pulmonary function tests (PFT).* In primary pulmonary hypertension, lung function tests usually show a modest decrease in both total lung capacity and diffusing capacity for carbon monoxide, but their principal value is (in conjunction with the chest radiograph) in excluding significant intrinsic lung disease as a cause of the elevated vascular resistance. Arterial gas analysis almost invariably reveals hypoxaemia, but hypocarbia may also be present by the time of presentation.

*Electro/Echocardiogram.* In both primary and secondary disease, the ECG characteristically shows right axis deviation, right ventricular hypertrophy and right ventricular strain. Echocardiography not only shows right ventricular enlargement with a normal or small left ventricular end-diastolic diameter, but also permits the non-invasive estimation of pulmonary artery pressure from the regurgitant jet across the tricuspid valve.

*Catheter studies.* Right heart catheterisation offers more direct and accurate assessment of the severity of disease and using thermodilution estimates of cardiac output, enables PVR to be calculated in the manner described above. Radioisotope perfusion lung scanning should be performed to exclude thromboembolic disease of the major pulmonary vessels. A high proportion of patients have abnormal scans, but only a minority show discrete defects. It has been suggested that ventilation/perfusion scanning can differentiate between the plexogenic and thromboembolic forms of the disease, but pulmonary angiography remains the diagnostic procedure of choice and should be carried out in all cases where the diagnosis is in doubt.

---

> **Box 8.4   Poor prognostic features in primary pulmonary hypertension**
>
> Mixed venous oxygen saturation > 63% (3-year survival > 55%)
> Elevated right atrial pressure
> Cardiac index < 2.0 l/min/m$^2$

---

This investigation has been used to identify poor prognostic features in patients with primary pulmonary hypertension, which appear to be a mixed venous oxygen saturation < 63%, cardiac index < 2.0 l/min/m$^2$ and high right atrial pressures (Box 8.4). Management policies depend to a certain extent on these variables.

*Tissue diagnosis.* The value of open lung biopsy remains contentious. On the one hand it is a potentially hazardous procedure and (equally importantly) may compromise subsequent selection for heart-lung transplantation. On the other hand, primary pulmonary hypertension appears to be a heterogeneous condition in both histology and the individual patientís response to therapy. However, not only is histological differentiation between subtypes imperfect for the reasons mentioned; but histological subtype seems to be a poor predictor of response to treatment. Nevertheless, tissue diagnosis may be useful in differentiating cases of pulmonary veno-occlusive disease (for which no medical therapy exists), rare cases of vasculitis and unsuspected interstitial fibrotic lung disease.

## Therapeutics

### Primary pulmonary hypertension (Fig. 8.1)

Conducting satisfactory controlled trials of therapeutic interventions in primary pulmonary hypertension is hampered by the rarity of the condition and the variability of its natural history. Despite this, it is generally accepted that treatment with anti-inflammatory drugs, such as corticosteroids and oxygen (except for the

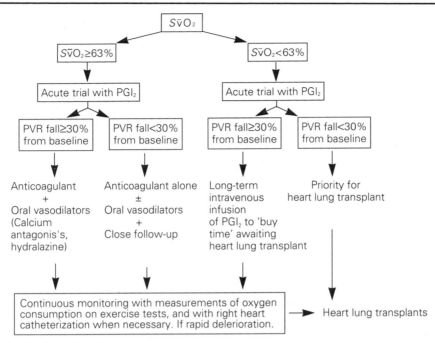

**Fig. 8.1** Practical assessment and management in primary pulmonary hypertension. Reproduced from Benetar et al 1986 by kind permission of the editor of the British Journal of Diseases of the Chest.

relief of severe hypoxaemia) is ineffective. Indeed, recent work suggests that the contribution of hypoxic pulmonary vasoconstriction may not be significant in determining the severity of disease. The remaining therapies employed include anticoagulation, vasodilators and more recently heart–lung transplantation.

*Anticoagulation.* The rationale for anticoagulation is based on the common association between primary pulmonary hypertension and histological evidence of microthrombotic lesions. Their role in pathogenesis is controversial and to date no well-designed prospective trial has demonstrated long-term anticoagulation to have a beneficial effect on mortality. Nevertheless, oral warfarin sufficient to maintain the prothrombin time at 2.0–2.5 times normal has been associated with improved survival following the retrospective analysis of data obtained from patients awaiting heart–lung transplantation.

*Vasodilator therapy. Acute* (Box 8.5). The potential benefits of vasodilator therapy

patients with primary pulmonary hypertension are several, including improved pulmonary haemodynamics, enhanced right ventricular function and increased oxygen delivery. Early work showed that a proportion of patients responded in this manner to the infusion of priscoline and acetylcholine, the potential benefits being reinforced by reports that acute vasoconstriction might progress eventually to fixed obstruction.

---

**Box 8.5  Acute vasodilator trial in primary pulmonary hypertension**

Prostacyclin (1–10 ng/kg/min infused via a pulmonary artery catheter)
or
Adenosine (5 mg/ml) infused via a pulmonary artery catheter (0.001–0.05 mg/kg bodyweight per min)

Positive response = > 20% fall in pulmonary vascular resistance

Conversely, vasodilator therapy has potentially adverse effects, including systemic hypotension and increased perfusion of poorly ventilated areas of lung, thereby impairing gas exchange and oxygen delivery. Numerous vasodilators have been used; including adrenergic antagonists (phentolamine, prazosin), parasympathomimetic agents (acetylcholine), $\beta$-adrenergic agonists (isoproteronol), direct acting vasodilators (nitrates, hydralazine), calcium-channel blocking agents (nifedipine, diltiazem, verapamil), angiotensin converting enzyme inhibitors (captopril), prostaglandins (prostacyclin, $PGE_1$) and atrial natriuretic peptide. It is clearly important that the effects of vasodilator therapy should be carefully assessed under controlled conditions within the intensive care unit prior to the commencement of long-term therapy. Most authorities suggest that a fall in pulmonary artery pressure (of at least 10%) and a rise in cardiac output, leading to a fall in PVR of > 20%, are the ideal responses to such a therapeutic trial, although only a minority of patients respond in this manner. Furthermore, the lack of selectivity of most vasodilators used acutely can make such therapeutic trials hazardous, particularly in patients with 'fixed' pulmonary vasculature.

Intravenous therapies are the safest agents available for this purpose, being short acting and therefore quickly reversible. Prostacyclin (1–10 ng/kg/min infused via a pulmonary artery catheter) is the most commonly used drug in this respect. Long and Rubin have shown that of 100 patients with primary pulmonary hypertension tested with prostacyclin, none who failed to respond acutely with a fall in PVR subsequently proved responsive to any other vasodilator. Furthermore, all patients who responded to prostacyclin proved responsive to at least one other vasodilator. Adenosine (5 mg/ml) infused via a pulmonary artery catheter (0.001–0.05 mg/kg body weight per minute) has also been shown recently to be an effective and selective short-acting pulmonary vasodilator in these circumstances. In a group of eight patients with PPH, mean maximal percent fall in PVR

from baseline was 39%.

Patients who show the most marked haemodynamic benefits in such short-term trials also seem to display the most symptomatic improvement during chronic treatment. Although both adenosine and prostacyclin can only be administered intravenously and are unsuitable for long-term use, some centres have used chronic infusions of the latter (2.5–10 ng/kg/min depending upon the response of both pulmonary and systemic haemodynamics to acute infusion) as maintenance therapy in patients awaiting lung or heart–lung transplantation.

*Chronic* (Table 8.4). The long-term effects of the oral vasodilator therapies currently available on quality of life and survival are still unclear. Continued responsiveness to vasodilators has been confirmed in individual patients up to six years after starting therapy, but such optimism is tempered by the fact that most of the published trials include insufficient numbers of patients to be confident of the results. Furthermore, recent reports to the effect that withdrawal of long-term treatment does not invariably result in a subsequent rise in pulmonary artery pressure, have led to confusion regarding the beneficial effects of chronic therapy and speculation regarding the spontaneous variation in pulmonary haemodynamics observed in such patients.

The chronic vasodilators used most frequently at present are the calcium channel blockers. Both oral nifedipine (20 mg) or diltiazem (60 mg) for patients with resting tachycardia, have been used to define sub-groups of patients showing favourable acute responses in pulmonary haemodynamics. The drugs are administered in repeated hourly doses until a favourable response (> 20% fall in PVR) is achieved, or systemic hypotension or another intolerable side-effect stops further progression of the trial. Naturally, all patients need to be fully instrumented and carefully monitored in an intensive care environment during this procedure. Using oral, rather than intravenous preparations for acute trials of pulmonary vascular responsiveness is more hazardous, but both nifedipine and diltiazem can be subsequently administered orally in those patients who respond favourably.

In one of the most recent studies, patients who responded with a > 20% fall in PVR were treated with nifedipine or diltiazem in the maximum dose tolerated acutely for up to 5 years (mean daily dose for nifedipine 172 mg and for diltiazem 720 mg) and their survival compared with those who did not respond and also with an NIH registry cohort. After 5 years, 94% of the responders were still alive compared with 55% of non-responders. The survival of the responders was also significantly better than that of the NIH registry cohort. Results such as these are difficult to obtain for reasons outlined above, but suggest that high-dose therapy with calcium channel blockers in patients with primary pulmonary hypertension can improve long-term survival in those who respond with an acute fall in pulmonary vascular resistance. Importantly, warfarin therapy was associated with improved survival, particularly in the subset of patients who did not respond to the calcium channel blockers.

*Heart–lung transplantation.* To date, the success of medical therapy in improving the prognosis of primary pulmonary hypertension has been limited. Heart–lung transplantation is therefore increasingly performed on the understanding that the disease is otherwise rapidly fatal and patients surviving the perioperative period (approximately 66%) have a marked improvement in quality of life and a relatively good prognosis. The major long-term complication of this procedure is obliterative bronchiolitis consequent upon sub-acute rejection. Cost, supply of donors and the limited number of centres also restricts the availability of this approach. Patient selection is difficult because primary pulmonary hypertension is a heterogeneous condition with variable survival, and precise indicators of prognosis in individual patients do not exist.

*Management summary: primary pulmonary hypertension* (Fig. 8.1). Once the diagnosis is established, all patients with primary pul-

monary hypertension should be subjected to an acute trial of vasodilator therapy (using prostacyclin or adenosine) whilst fully instrumented and monitored in an intensive care environment. Those who respond favourably (> 20% fall in PVR) and have good prognostic features (mixed venous oxygen saturation > 63%, cardiac index > 2 l/min/m², low right atrial pressures) should be treated with the maximum dose of oral calcium channel antagonist (nifedipine, diltiazem) they can tolerate, given oral anticoagulants and reviewed regularly with exercise testing and re-catheterisation at yearly intervals. Those who do not have a favourable acute response (< 20% fall in PVR), but have good prognostic features should be anticoagulated and followed in a similar fashion. Both groups should be referred for assessment for heart–lung or lung transplantation if they deteriorate clinically or haemodynamically.

Patients with poor prognostic features, but showing a favourable response to acute vasodilators should be given either oral calcium antagonists or (if available and practical) long-term infused prostacyclin to 'buy time' whilst being assessed for transplantation. Finally, those with a poor response to vasodilators and poor prognostic features should be given a priority for transplantation if suitable.

### Secondary pulmonary hypertension

Secondary pulmonary hypertension is diagnosed by the demonstration of an elevated PVR in the presence of cardiopulmonary disease. Pulmonary artery catheterisation is carried out relatively rarely in this group of patients. A positive history of chronic chest disease coupled with clinical evidence of pulmonary hypertension and radiographic and ECG/echocardiographic confirmation of elevated PVR is usually considered sufficient to make the diagnosis. Poor prognostic features identified have therefore been clinical (see 'Prognosis'). Therapeutic options are limited and depend to a certain extent upon the underlying disease (e.g. bronchodilators in COPD).

Many are discussed elsewhere (see chronic respiratory failure).

*Oxygen therapy.* The benefits and application of oxygen therapy in hypoxic cor pulmonale have been described elsewhere. It has been suggested that the poor prognosis of this condition is related to the severity of the pulmonary hypertension, although recent histopathological studies have not always supported this contention. Nevertheless, the reduction in mortality consequent upon the advent of long-term domiciliary oxygen therapy (LTO$_2$) is associated with the prevention in the progressive rise in PVR seen in this condition. This has also provided the rationale for the attempted use of pulmonary vasodilators in cor pulmonale; a therapy that might improve prognosis per se, or reduce the dependence upon LTO$_2$.

*Vasodilator therapy* (Table 8.4). Evidence suggests that oxygen is relatively ineffective in actually reducing PVR in secondary pulmonary hypertension. Many therapeutic trials of vasodilators have therefore been carried out in an effort to replace or augment what is onerous and expensive therapy. Initial success with agents such as tolazoline, phentolamine, nitrates, nitroprusside and diazoxide was limited by their routes of administration and unacceptable side-effects. Oral hydralazine produced beneficial effects in some, but not all studies. Other agents used include prostaglandin E1 derivatives, captopril, pirbuterol and α-methyl dopa. More recently, the calcium antagonists nifedipine and verapamil have been shown to inhibit hypoxic pulmonary vasoconstriction in animal models. The results in patients with COPD have, however, been conflicting. In similar fashion to trials in patients with primary pulmonary hypertension, most drugs used have had a bigger effect on the systemic circulation. Cardiac output often increases and pulmonary artery pressure may fall or more commonly, remain unchanged. In some cases the vasodilation in areas of poor ventilation increases ventilation ($\dot{V}$) – perfusion ($\dot{Q}$) mismatch thus lowering arterial oxygen tension, although the increase in cardiac output may

**Table 8.4  Vasodilator agents that have been used in the acute assessment and/or chronic management of either primary or secondary pulmonary hypertension**

| | |
|---|---|
| α-adrenergic antagonists | Phentolamine Prazosin |
| Parasympathomimetic agents | Acetylcholine |
| β-adrenergic agonists | Isoproteronol |
| Direct-acting vasodilator | Nitrates Hydralazine |
| Calcium-channel-blockers | Nifedipine Diltiazem |
| Angiotensin converting enzyme inhibitors (ACE) | Captopril |
| Prostacyclin | Prostacyclin (PGE1) |
| Atrial naturetic hormone Adenosine | |

maintain oxygen delivery. Long-term placebo-controlled trials are required to assess precisely what benefit, if any, such drugs may have in this group of patients. The prognosis in secondary pulmonary hypertension is complicated by issues unrelated to the pulmonary circulation, such as lung function. In these circumstances it is possibly not surprising that the acute haemodynamic effects induced by a variety of agents do not appear to predict changes seen after only a few weeks' therapy. Furthermore, the high mortality associated with cor pulmonale is such that recruiting adequate numbers of patients is difficult. Repeated measurements of PVR need to be made and at present this can only be achieved by invasive means.

*Management summary: secondary pulmonary hypertension.* The current management is determined by the therapy most appropriate for the underlying condition. LTO$_2$ should be prescribed for those meeting current criteria (see chronic respiratory failure). There is no place for vasodilator therapy at present.

## Prognosis

The prognosis for pulmonary hypertension as a whole is poor. The commonest modes of death are right heart failure and sudden death. A few patients with primary pulmonary hypertension do enjoy long-term survival and spontaneous remissions have been reported. Data from Stanford in 90 patients referred for heart–lung transplantation (of whom 18 underwent surgery), suggests 5- and 10-year survival rates of 37% and 15% respectively. These patients had a mean age of 29.8 years at diagnosis and represent a selected series in terms of age and the fact that all had been considered sufficiently unwell (New York Heart Association Grade III, IV) to be placed on the waiting list for transplantation. Other series include that of Fuster and colleagues which reported a median survival of 1.9 years in 112 patients who survived cardiac catheterisation. Precise indicators are not available to identify patients likely to become long-term survivors. Parameters of right heart function appear to correlate best with prognosis and evidence of elevated right atrial pressure at diagnosis is a poor prognostic sign. A low pulmonary artery oxygen saturation and low cardiac output at diagnosis are also said to correlate highly with reduced survival.

In patients with pulmonary hypertension secondary to hypoxic lung disease, the development of hypoxic cor pulmonale (clinical and ECG evidence of right heart failure in the absence of congenital or acquired myocardial disease) in association with peripheral oedema carries a 5-year mortality approaching 66% (see also chronic respiratory failure).

## Therapeutic prospects in pulmonary hypertension

Considerable advances in the understanding of pulmonary vascular control, particularly under hypoxic conditions and following lung injury, have highlighted the importance of the endothelium in vascular regulation. It is likely that future manipulation of the pulmonary circulation will depend upon endothelially-derived relaxant and constricting factors (EDRF, EDCF). EDRF is almost certainly nitric oxide (NO), which has already been shown in pilot studies to be effective in reducing PVR selectively when administered by inhalation to patients with primary pulmonary hypertension.

Pulmonary hypertension remains a poorly understood condition; heterogeneous in its natural history, histology and response to therapy. In particular, the rarity of primary pulmonary hypertension and the absence of a suitable animal model have hindered the establishment of sufficient well-controlled studies of potential therapeutic interventions, but current investigations give hope that vasodilator therapy may prove beneficial for some. Meanwhile, heart–lung transplantation provides an alternative solution for a few patients with this devastating disease. As has been stated elsewhere, the principal cause of cor pulmonale is COPD, the incidence of which would be greatly diminished if cigarette smoking were to cease.

## THROMBOEMBOLIC DISEASE

### Epidemiology and definition

It has been estimated that in the USA 300 000 patients are hospitalised and 50 000 die each year due to thromboembolic disease. In the UK an estimated 20 000 die each year in hospital as a result of pulmonary embolus PE and 40 000 have non-fatal episodes. It is important to emphasise that PE is not a disease in itself, but rather a complication of deep venous thrombosis (DVT). Equally important is the recognition that over 90% of pulmonary emboli arise from thrombi in the deep veins of the lower extremities, although not all pose equal risks. Thus, thrombi confined to the calf are usually small and even if untreated are associated with excellent clinical outcome. Lastly, available data suggest that 75–95% of patients dying from PE die within the first few hours of the embolic event. Most deaths occurring after the first few hours are due to recurrent emboli.

| Table 8.5   Diagnosis of deep vein thrombosis |
| --- |
| **Proven:** |
| Contrast venography |
| Impedence plethysmography |
| Radiofibrinogen leg scanning |
| **Under evaluation:** |
| Radiovenography |
| Doppler flow |
| Doppler/ultrasound ('Duplex') |

**Box 8.6   Prevention and therapy of DVT**

**Effective DVT prophylaxis includes:**

Low-dose s/c heparin (5000 8–12 hrly)
Full-length anti-embolism stockings
Intermittent pneumatic compression

**Treatment of DVT:**

Heparin s/c twice daily (30–35 000 u/24h, to keep
KCCT 1.5–2.5 times normal)
or, continuous infusion i.v. Heparin to same limits
continued for 5 days with:
Warfarin started on day 1 (dose to maintain PT
between 2 and 3 times normal) for 12 weeks

The therapeutic implications of these facts are several. Firstly, the management of DVT assumes equal significance to that of PE. Secondly, those DVTs confined to the calf and presenting with easily detectable clinical signs of redness, pain and swelling are not necessarily those to worry about, and thirdly most embolic *deaths* occur so rapidly that neither appropriate diagnostic nor therapeutic measures can be instituted.

# Deep venous thrombosis (DVT)

Factors predisposing to DVT formation are local trauma to the vessel wall, hypercoagulability and blood stasis. Although a number of well-recognised haematological abnormalities are associated with a higher incidence of disease, such as deficiencies of anti thrombin III and the presence of lupus anticoagulant, other conditions including recent surgery, the contraceptive pill, indwelling venous catheters, advanced age, cancer and low cardiac output, all contribute to thrombus formation. 35–50% of patients with DVTs suffer eventually from pulmonary embolus although the clinical sequelae are variable. DVTs confined to the calf have a much reduced incidence of embolism.

## Diagnosis

A diagnosis based on clinical grounds is almost always inaccurate. Although many other inves-

tigations have been devised, including impedance plethysmograph, isotope-labelled fibrinogen uptake and venous doppler techniques, the venogram remains the gold-standard by which all others are judged (Table 8.5).

## *Prevention and therapy* (Box 8.6)

Prevention of DVT of the lower extremities will automatically reduce the frequency of embolism. As most patients subsequently developing a fatal PE die within hours, no treatment modality can have the same effect as prevention, which involves identifying the patients at risk and adopting prophylactic options. The former include any individual in whom some combination of venous stasis, vessel injury and coagulation changes may exist. Effective prophylaxis includes the application of intermittent venous compression devices to the lower limbs during surgery, passive compression stockings, and anticoagulant therapy (Table 8.6). Low-dose heparin (5000 units subcutaneously 8–12 hourly, via pre-loaded syringes) starting at the time of risk and carrying on until the patient is ambulatory is extremely effective. Small doses of warfarin (1–2 mg) prior to surgery are also effective in preventing DVT even in high-risk patients. The identification of any proximal DVT is justification for anticoagulation with heparin, administered either subcutaneously or preferably by infusion and with a dose adjusted

**Table 8.6   Diagnosis of pulmonary embolus: probability**

| Probability of pulmonary embolism on basis of lung scan | Clinical assessment of probability of pulmonary embolism | | |
|---|---|---|---|
| | Low (%) | Medium (%) | High (%) |
| *Perfusion scan* | | | |
| Low | | | |
|   Subsegmental defect(s) | 1 | 2 (10) | 10 (25) |
| Medium | | | |
|   Segmental defect(s) | 10 | 25 (75) | 65 (85) |
| High | | | |
|   Lobar defect(s) | 25 | 55 (90) | 85 (95) |
| *Ventilation/perfusion scan* | | | |
| Low | | | |
|   Matching defect(s) | 2 | 2 | 2 |
| Medium | | | |
|   Mismatched subsegmental defect(s) | 1 | 3 (22) | 40 (70) |
| High | | | |
|   Mismatched segmental or lobar defect(s) | 55 | 80 (95) | 95 (100) |

Figures in parentheses relate to multiple scan defects in each category (Reproduced from Benatar et al)

according to the Kaolin-Cephalin Clotting Time (KCCT). Animal data suggest that if this regimen is adopted, venous thrombi do not grow and the incidence of recurrent venous thrombosis and PEs is reduced. The only complication of this therapy is haemorrhage, unfortunately not predicted by the level of anticoagulation, and thrombocytopenia. A minimum of 5 days' i.v. therapy should be followed by oral therapy with Warfarin. Warfarin anticoagulation is monitored by prothrombin time (PT), usually maintained at approximately twice the normal level. In patients in whom there is a substantial risk of haemorrhage, such as following major trauma or brain/spinal cord injury, monitoring and prophylaxis may be impossible. The only alternative therapy at present widely adopted (mainly in the USA) in these circumstances is the insertion of a vena caval filter. Current data suggest that the recurrence of venous thrombosis is likely for at least 3 and possibly 6 months and the duration of anticoagulation should reflect this although the optimal duration of

therapy has not been determined by any therapeutic trial. Clearly, the continued presence of risk factors will influence this to a certain extent. Some authorities in the USA continue therapy until impedance plethysmography has returned to normal.

Thrombolytic therapy (streptokinase and tissue plasminogen activator) can lead to a more rapid resolution of venous thrombi and the restoration of more normal anatomy, but whether this leads to lower recurrence rates or a reduced length of hospital stay is unclear. Furthermore, many patients with DVTs are unsuitable for fibrinolytic therapy because of recent surgery or trauma. Some centres, again in the USA, have confined their use of such agents to severe ileofemoral thromboses where the outcome with standard heparin therapy is poor.

## Pulmonary embolus

The clinical consequences of pulmonary embolus are varied, depending upon the extent of the pulmonary vascular tree that is occluded, the patient's pre-existing cardiopulmonary status and the subsequent release of humeral factors such as prostaglandins, serotonin and thromboxane. The treatment of pulmonary embolus follows the same general principles as for DVT, but in order to determine precise therapeutic strategies, patients with thromboembolic disease may be divided into four groups:

### Acute minor pulmonary embolus

Small quantities of thrombus lodging in the pulmonary capillary bed may be asymptomatic or can result in pleuritic chest pain, dyspnoea, cough or haemoptysis. Physical examination may be normal or reveal relatively non-specific findings such as tachycardia or a pleural rub. Pulmonary infarction only occurs in these circumstances if oedema consequent upon obstruction to the pulmonary artery compresses the bronchial arterial blood supply.

*Diagnosis.* Unless infarction sufficient to cause mismatched abnormalities on an isotope ventilation ($\dot{V}$) – perfusion ($\dot{Q}$) scan occur, diagnosis is difficult. A chest radiograph is essential for correct interpretation of the $\dot{V}/\dot{Q}$ scan. Perfusion defects in the presence of radiographic abnormalities at the same site cannot be ascribed to an embolus with any degree of confidence. The need for angiography following acute minor PE is still a matter of debate. Broadly speaking, a high probability of PE clinically together with a high probability on $\dot{V}/\dot{Q}$ scanning suggests that treatment can be instituted immediately. A low clinical probability with an abnormal $\dot{V}/\dot{Q}$ scan is an indication for angiograms in order to identify the 40% or so of such patients with emboli (Table 8.6).

### Acute massive pulmonary embolus

Acute massive pulmonary embolus results from the occlusion of more than 50% of the pulmonary vascular tree and causes severe respiratory distress and circulatory collapse.

*Diagnosis.* There is usually profound arterial hypoxaemia, hypocapnea, a metabolic acidosis and (in a minority of patients) electrocardiographic evidence of severe right heart strain (the classical 'S1, Q3, T3' pattern). The chest radiograph may show non-specific features of patchy oligaemia with arterial dilatation. Ideally, pulmonary angiography should be performed to confirm the diagnosis. Pulmonary artery pressures may be moderately elevated, or can be low if the right ventricle has failed following the sudden increase in afterload. Patients with the gradual onset of chronic thromboembolic disease may have marked elevations in pulmonary artery pressure, but in those where the degree of pulmonary arterial obstruction is prolonged and severe, syncope or death may ensue.

### Chronic thromboembolic disease

The sub-classification of unexplained pulmonary hypertension into three pathological categories represented an attempt to differentiate between plexogenic arteriopathy and thromboembolic aetiologies. It is impossible to differentiate these two on clinical grounds alone, although in the only large series to be published, patients with primary plexogenic arteriopathy had significantly higher mean pulmonary artery pressures at presentation than did those with chronic thromboembolic disease. Survival from the time of diagnosis was poor in both groups and was not significantly correlated with any measured haemodynamic parameter. Whether or not a distinction might be desirable therapeutically remains unclear. Although the current tendency is to anticoagulate all patients, no prospective controlled trials have been carried out to determine the effects of such therapy on survival.

### Therapy in pulmonary embolus

Beyond instigating supportive measures such as oxygen therapy and analgesia, the major therapeutic options for pulmonary embolus are as follows:

*Heparin.* Heparin accelerates the action of thrombin III and prevents further fibrin deposi-

**Table 8.7 Thrombolytic therapy in acute massive pulmonary embolus**

**Therapy**

Streptokinase (250 000 u infused via a peripheral venous catheter over 30 min followed by 100 000 u per hour for 20 h) or (if streptokinase is contraindicated):
Tissue plasminogen activator (50 mg over 2 h followed by 50 mg over 5 h if the rate of resolution is poor)

Arterial oxygen saturations should begin to improve within an hour of commencing therapy and considerable benefit is usually apparent within 3–4 hours. Any patient with AMPE who continues to deteriorate at that time should be considered for surgery

**Contraindications**

Recent (< 2 weeks) major surgery
Cerebrovascular accident (< 2–3 months)
Bleeding diathesis or active peptic ulceration

tion, allowing the endogenous fibrinolytic system to lyse existing clot. There has been only one randomised trial comparing heparin with placebo after PE which was stopped after only 35 patients were enrolled because of a markedly increased mortality in the placebo group. The investigators concluded that heparin may not reduce the immediate mortality of PE, but probably reduced deaths due to further emboli. Despite such evidence, many clinicians continue to use heparin alone after massive PE when at best it can only prevent further emboli whilst the patient's own fibrinolytic system dissolves the obstructing thrombus.

*Thrombolysis* (Table 8.7). Intravenous streptokinase and urokinase were shown to be better than heparin alone in hastening the resolution of acute massive pulmonary embolus in the early 1970s, but even now such agents are used infrequently. Although mortality has been shown to be lower with thrombolysis than with heparin alone, no comparative trial has yet shown a significant difference in mortality. Despite this lack of statistical proof of prognostic benefit, achieving a more rapid resolution of

pulmonary emboli would seem to be desirable, since haemodynamic disturbance would otherwise be prolonged and further emboli, should they occur, would have a smaller effect. Secondly, potentially dangerous ileofemoral thrombi may be incidentally lysed. Thrombolytic agents such as streptokinase (250 000 units infused over 30 min followed by 100 000 units per hour for 24 h) administered via a peripheral venous catheter, or tissue plasminogen activator (50 mg over 2 h followed by 50 mg over 5 h if the rate of resolution is poor) have been shown conclusively to hasten the resolution of pulmonary emboli. Contraindications include recent (< 2 weeks) major surgery, cerebrovascular accident (< 2–3 months), bleeding diathesis or active peptic ulceration. Thrombolytic agents may be safely given and their effects monitored in non-specialist centres, but a number of questions remain unanswered. Which agent (streptokinase, tissue plasminogen activator, urokinase) is superior is still not clear and comparative trials using comparable doses of each have not been performed. Whether large boluses of streptokinase are as effective as infusions over 24 hours is also unknown. However, as these agents remain underused, it is probably more important at present for the clinician to ensure that patients receive any available thrombolytic drug quickly in doses known to be effective.

*Surgical management.* The debate regarding surgical embolectomy versus thrombolytic therapy following massive PE has been strong since the latter first became available in the mid 1970s. Certainly in those patients too ill to undergo thrombolysis or with specific contraindications (see below), pulmonary embolectomy in skilled hands offers an effective alternative treatment. In one large series, 70% of patients treated surgically survived, largely without morbidity, even though many had suffered from episodes of cardiac arrest.

*Inferior vena caval interruption.* Residual thrombus almost always remains in the deep veins of the lower limb after PE occurs. Attempts have been made to prevent recurrence

| Table 8.8 Treatment of pulmonary embolus | |
|---|---|
| **Acute minor** | **Acute massive** |
| Oxygen | Oxygen |
| Analgesia | Volume resuscitation |
| Heparin, warfarin | Inotropes |
| | Thrombolysis |
| | (Embolectomy), warfarin |

by surgical interruption or plication of the inferior vena cava (IVC), although the insertion of 'umbrella' or filtration devices percutaneously is now more popular. Their effectiveness in reducing recurrence following PE has never been proven in controlled trials and recurrent emboli are in any case uncommon (< 10%). Furthermore, in the absence of continuing risk factors, progression to chronic thromboembolic pulmonary hypertension is rare. However, for those patients in whom anticoagulation is contraindicated or who have recurrent emboli despite such therapy, insertion of an IVC filter should be considered.

### Management summary: pulmonary embolus
(Table 8.8)

A clear history is required, both of the patient's individual symptoms and of any risk factors. A chest radiograph, ECG and radionuclide ($\dot{V}/\dot{Q}$) lung scan should be performed. Subsequent management depends upon the degree of haemodynamic disturbance the PE has induced.

*Acute minor pulmonary embolus.* Patients with no haemodynamic disturbance should be given symptomatic relief with simple analgesics and oxygen. For those with evidence of pulmonary emboli on $\dot{V}/\dot{Q}$ scanning, heparin should be given sufficient to keep the KCCT at 1.5–2.5 times normal (e.g. 100 units/kg loading dose, followed by 1000–2000 units/h). This will not speed the resolution of the embolus, but prevents further propagation of clot in the deep veins whilst the endogenous fibrinolytic system works. Low molecular weight subcutaneous heparins may be easier to administer, have a

longer half-life than the i.v. preparation, and have a more favourable antithrombotic to haemorrhagic ratio, but the risk of bleeding may be greater. Oral anticoagulation with warfarin in the manner described above (see management of DVT), started after 48 hours, is recommended. The duration of both therapies should be as described for DVT. Whether 3 months' oral anticoagulation is really necessary in these circumstances remains unclear, although there is some evidence of increased recurrence if therapy is continued for only 1 month. The isotope lung scan can be a useful adjunct to guide the duration of therapy and long-term protective anticoagulation may be justifiable if a significant perfusion defect remains even in the absence of risk factors or residual DVT.

*Acute massive pulmonary embolus.* As the principal problem is one of acute right ventricular failure, therapy is aimed at maintaining cardiac output by optimising filling pressures, the judicious use of inotropes, and the application of interventions aimed at relieving the obstruction to outflow. A central venous catheter is necessary to allow the administration of fluids and where thrombolytic therapy is to be used, a jugular approach is preferable. The introduction of pulmonary artery catheter of the thermodilution type is also desirable, to permit the measurement of cardiac output and to assess the effects of therapeutic interventions on PVR. Transcutaneous oximetry can also provide some indication of the efficacy of thrombolysis in relieving pulmonary arterial obstruction. If doubt exists regarding the diagnosis, pulmonary angiography or isotope scanning should be carried out. Thrombolyic therapy should then be instituted, or pulmonary embolectomy considered if the former is contraindicated. Streptokinase 250 000–600 000 units. as an intravenous loading dose administered with 100 mg hydrocortisone via the central venous/pulmonary artery catheter should be followed by a further 100 000 units per hour for 72 hours. Heparin anticoagulation for 3 days with the simultaneous administration of warfarin (see above) is recommended. Arterial oxygen saturations should begin to improve within an hour of commencing therapy and considerable benefit is usually apparent within 3–4 hours. Any patient with acute massive who continues to deteriorate at that time should be considered for surgery.

*Chronic thromboembolic disease.* The insidious nature of this condition means that it frequently presents late, at a stage where there is often little alternative to thromboendarterectomy or heart–lung/lung transplantation. Domiciliary oxygen may help symptomatically.

## ADULT RESPIRATORY DISTRESS SYNDROME

The adult respiratory distress syndrome (ARDS) is characterised by high permeability pulmonary oedema and refractory hypoxaemia. ARDS is associated with a wide variety of serious surgical and medical pathologies and carries a mortality approaching 60%, little changed from that reported when the condition was first described over 20 years ago. No effective therapeutic interventions have been developed and treatment remains almost entirely supportive in nature. Nevertheless, the condition has provoked a large amount of basic scientific and clinical research. ARDS is characterised by increased pulmonary vascular permeability secondary to endothelial cell damage, but there is increasing awareness that ARDS is a systemic condition and that not only the pulmonary vascular endothelium is involved. Therapies are therefore aimed at supporting all organ systems, not merely the lung. In view of the limited scope of this book, only the newer techniques of respiratory support and potential pharmacological interventions will be described.

### New approaches to ventilatory support

The conventional approach to the respiratory support of patients with ARDS involves administering tidal volume preset, controlled mandatory ventilation; the appropriate use of positive

end expiratory pressure (PEEP) and an inspiratory to expiratory (I:E) time ratio of less than one. The mandatory delivery of a preset tidal volume, regardless of the level of PEEP and the respiratory system compliance, may result in high peak and mean airway pressures (PIP, MAP), leading to haemodynamic compromise and the potential for barotrauma. Haemodynamic depression results from increased intrapleural pressure which reduces venous return and causes direct cardiac compression. Optimising cardiac performance and hence oxygen delivery, depends upon minimising this effect. The pressure rise is a consequence of the fractional transmission of airway pressure to the intrapleural space, which is attenuated to a certain extent in ARDS by decreased lung compliance. Barotrauma is a complex phenomenon and results not only in pneumothorax and pneumomediastinum, but also produces pulmonary interstitial emphysema in the perivascular and peribronchiolar regions. The main risk factor is thought to be high PIPs. Although no safe upper limit for PIP has been defined, a significant incidence of barotrauma can be expected at levels in excess of 50 cm $H_2O$. Furthermore, barotrauma resulting from high PIP may actually exacerbate the pulmonary pathology of ARDS and contribute to the ultimate disturbance of lung architecture associated with the syndrome. Lung pathology in ARDS is characterised by diffuse alveolar damage in which there is widespread micro-atelectasis resulting in a diffuse reduction in the size of alveolar spaces. Such sites represent areas of $\dot{V}/\dot{Q}$ mismatch and explain the situation frequently encountered in ARDS whereby $CO_2$ clearance can be improved by regional hyperventilation of the functioning lung units, but oxygenation remains virtually impossible. It is now recognised that whatever ventilatory mode is used, oxygenation can be improved by the recruitment of unstable alveoli and by preventing their subsequent collapse. Originally, this was thought best achieved by the application of positive end expiratory pressure (PEEP); which, when used in conjunction with conven-

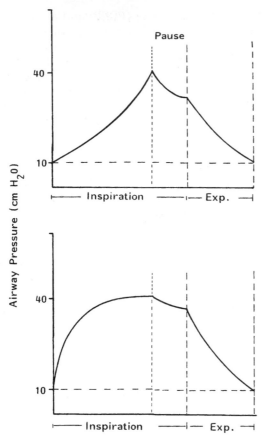

**Fig. 8.2** Inverse ratio ventilation and airway pressure-release ventilation.

tional ventilation, is often accompanied by unacceptably high PIPs or haemodynamic impairment.

## New modes of ventilation (Fig. 8.2)

The strategy behind new approaches to ventilation is best summarised as aggressive alveolar recruitment and the maintenance of alveolar volume, avoiding high PIPs and maintaining adequate $CO_2$ clearance. Inverse ratio ventilation (IRV) represents a variant conventional ventilation in which I:E ratios of greater than 1:1 are applied. The technique has been used widely and with good results in neonatal units, but until recently there have been few reports of

its use in ARDS. The prolonged application of inspiratory positive pressure may recruit collapsed alveoli and the brief period of expiration, although adequate for $CO_2$ clearance, may retard expiration sufficiently to keep these alveoli above their closing volume. In volume-controlled inverse ratio ventilation (VC-IRV), a preset tidal volume is delivered with each breath, regardless of the end expiratory state of the respiratory system. The attraction of this technique lies in the combination of a predictable tidal volume with a rise in mean airway pressures (and hence oxygenation), unassociated with a rise in PIP. However, there is considerable potential for air trapping and 'stacking' of consecutive breaths if expiratory time is not optimised, thus leading to ever-increasing lung volumes and PIP in what is by definition a non-compliant respiratory system. Such a system of ventilation is unforgiving and although it is possible to introduce a safety-oriented peak-cycling pressure, this is accompanied by a decrease in tidal volume and therefore reduces effective alveolar ventilation. During pressure-controlled inverse ratio ventilation (PC-IRV), gas is delivered at a constant, preset PIP for the desired inspiratory time. The inspiratory flow profile depends upon the pressure gradient established between the ventilator and the alveoli and is thus maximal in the early part of inspiration when PIP is reached. As the pressure gradient declines, the inspiratory flow decelerates in an exponential fashion. A key element of this approach is the initiation of the subsequent breath prior to the cessation of expiratory flow, preventing the lung from falling to its functional residual capacity and preventing alveolar de-recruitment. In this context the tidal volume cannot be preset and is greatly influenced by the compliance of the respiratory system, making the measurement of expired gas volumes mandatory.

The use of high frequency jet ventilation (HFJV) in ARDS initially proved disappointing. Early studies suggested that significant improvements in oxygenation could be achieved only at the expense of increases in PIP and diminished cardiac output and that jet

| Table 8.9 | Extracorporeal gas exchange |
|-----------|------------------------------|
| ECGE | Extracorporeal gas exchange, the blanket term for all techniques of extracorporeal support. |
| ECMO | Extracorporeal membrane oxygenation; oxygenation is the prime objective of this technique, the transfer of carbon dioxide being a secondary effect. |
| $ECCO_2R$ | Extracorporeal carbon dioxide removal; removal of $CO_2$ is the primary aim, thereby reducing the requirement for conventional mechanical ventilatory support. |
| $P/TECCO_2R$ | Extracorporeal carbon dioxide removal may be partial ($PECCO_2R$) or total ($TECCO_2R$) depending upon the blood flow rate and the area of the gas exchanging membrane. |

## Extracorporeal respiratory support

The aim of extracorporeal gas exchange (ECGE) in ARDS is to adequately oxygenate the patient via a synthetic gas permeable membrane, thus preventing further tissue hypoxia and allowing the lung to 'rest' and undergo spontaneous repair without suffering from the barotrauma that is frequently the consequence of conventional mechanical ventilation. Extracorporeal membrane oxygenation (ECMO) is an established and valuable technique in the neonatal respiratory distress syndrome and was pioneered in ARDS in 1972. Disappointingly, subsequent controlled trials comparing ECMO to conventional ventilation in respiratory failure failed to show any increase in survival. Nevertheless, recent studies using a modified form of ECGE, termed extracorporeal carbon dioxide removal ($ECCO_2R$, Table 8.9), have shown survival rates of up to 50%. These encouraging results coupled with improvements in vascular access, membrane technology and anticoagulant pharmacology have led to a resurgence of interest in extracorporeal support for respiratory failure.

ventilation using frequencies around 100 breaths per minute only afforded significant advantages to patients with bronchopulmonary fistulae. The technique employs the principle of recruiting alveoli that are subsequently prevented from collapsing by the obligate PEEP that is consequent upon the short expiratory time and interest has recently been growing in using HFJV at ultra high frequencies, in the range 5–7 Hz. There have been suggestions that U-HFJV may actually reduce mean airway pressures when compared with conventional techniques and the results of randomised, prospective, controlled trials in patients with ARDS are in progress.

## Pharmacological intervention in ARDS

The commonest causes of lung injury in ARDS can be divided into two group: those that directly damage the lung and those in which a remote disease process results in ARDS, presumably through the action of inflammatory mediators (Box 8.7). It seems possible that iden-

| Box 8.7  Common causes of ARDS | |
|--------------------------------|---|
| **Pulmonary** | **Non-pulmonary** |
| Pneumonia: aspiration<br>　　　　　bacterial<br>Pulmonary contusion<br>Inhalation of toxic gases<br>Drug toxicity | Major trauma<br>Multiple blood transfusions<br>Pancreatitis<br>Amniotic fluid embolus<br>Fat embolus |

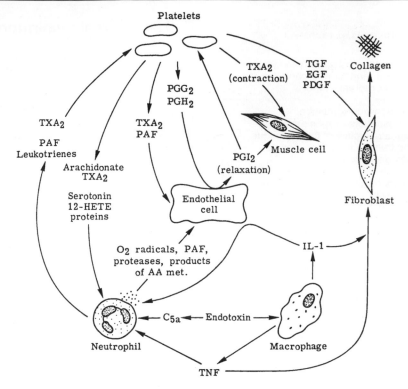

**Fig. 8.3** Interaction of neutrophils and vascular endothelial cells. Only recently has the significance of the endothelial cell in vascular control been appreciated. The release of endothelially derived relaxant and constricting factors (EDRF, EDCF) together with vasodilator prostaglandins (PG) may have important physiological consequences as neutrophils pass through the endothelial barrier.

tical mediators directly damage the alveolar capillary membrane when released locally, for example during pneumonia. Identifying these substances, their mechanisms of release, action and interaction therefore holds the key to understanding the pathophysiology of ARDS and thus developing effective therapeutic interventions (Figs 8.3, 8.4). Sepsis is a systemic insult resulting in panendothelial damage, cardiovascular dysfunction and ultimately MOF, which includes ARDS in 25–30% of cases. Recent reports which have described patients fulfilling the criteria for the sepsis syndrome with no demonstrable focus of infection suggest that uncontrolled activation of mediators of inflammation regardless of cause can reproduce clinical sepsis. Animal studies support this contention. An identical phenomenon has been described in patients with ARDS in whom

rigorous efforts were made to exclude infection. A model of interactions between some mediators thought to contribute to acute lung injury associated with sepsis is shown in Figures 8.3 and 8.4.

## New approaches to pharmacotherapy (Box 8.8)

### Steroids

Steroid therapy has been advocated for patients at risk from ARDS and those detected early in the course of the disease on the basis of favourable reports from non-randomised trials. A prospective study by Schumer also suggested that steroids reduced the mortality rate in septic shock from 38.4% to 10.5%. Nevertheless, two large randomised, controlled, prospective

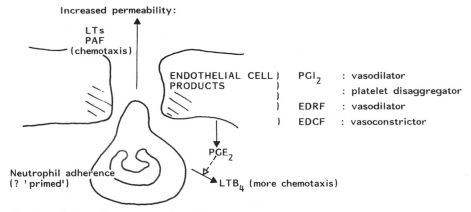

**Fig. 8.4** Schematic representation of the possible consequences of neutrophil activation by the cytokines tumour necrosis factor (TNF) and interleukin (IL). Note the redundancy built into the system, such that if one pathway to endothelial damage is blocked, another may produce the same end result.

studies in established ARDS failed to show any benefit from corticosteroid therapy and suggested that mortality in patients with sepsis may even be increased. Steroids have been used recently in patients recovering from ARDS who then developed the signs of sepsis with no identifiable source. Results from this study and isolated case reports in similar patients suggest that further trials of steroids in the late phase of ARDS are warranted.

### Neutralisation of the effects of endotoxin/ LPS1

Two large trials have been published recently describing the effects of monoclonal antibodies

---

> **Box 8.8  New approaches to pharmacotherapy in ARDS**
>
> Steroids
> Neutralisation of the effects of
> endotoxin/LPS1
> Modulation of the cytokine response
> Non-steroidal anti-inflammatory drugs
> (NSAID)
> Prostaglandin
> Anti oxidants
> Manipulation of the L-arginine pathway
> Pentoxifylline
> Surfactant

---

to endotoxin core glycoprotein in human sepsis syndrome. Both demonstrated advantages in terms of survival and resolution of system failures only in patient subsets. E5, a murine IgM antibody, significantly decreased mortality in patients with gram-negative sepsis with no evidence of circulatory shock. In this group (137 out of a total of 486), ARDS resolved in 4/10 patients who received E5 compared with 2/9 patients given placebo. By contrast, HA-1A, a human monoclonal IgM antibody, was found to be effective regardless of shock, but only in patients with proven gram-negative bacteraemia. Data specific to ARDS were not given, but in the group that responded all major morbidities (including ARDS) resolved within 7 days in 38/61 patients given HA-1A, compared with 26/62 given placebo. There were no significant side-effects attributable to either antibody. Problems that may inhibit the more widespread application of these novel treatments include their high cost and difficulties in identifying the minority (approximately one third) of patients likely to benefit from the therapy.

### Modulation of the cytokine response

It is theoretically possible to block the damaging effects of cytokines at a number of different levels (see Fig. 8.4). Although this exciting possibility has not yet been tried in vivo for the most part, animal studies have shown that when administered prophylactically, neutralising antibodies for TNF are protective against lethal endotoxaemia and bacteraemia, although only one study has demonstrated benefit when such antibodies were given after injury. A phase 1 study of a murine IgG monoclonal antibody to recombinant human TNF in patients with septic shock revealed no serious side-effects and results of a larger study examining therapeutic efficacy and effects on mortality are awaited.

Haemofiltration is a mainstay in the supportive therapy for MOF and ARDS, facilitating the correction of biochemical abnormalities and fluid balance, but recent studies have also suggested that high volume pumped veno-venous haemofiltration may be useful in removing mediators of sepsis. No trials have assessed the possible benefit from introducing haemofiltration in sepsis or ARDS earlier than indicated by traditional criteria. Future developments in this area may involve incorporation of antibodies or other materials known to bind cytokines into filtration membranes.

### Non-steroidal anti-inflammatory drugs (NSAIDs)

Clinical data on the use of NSAIDs in ARDS are scarce, although theoretically they should be of benefit in the late and established phases of ARDS. Indomethacin and meclofenamate have been shown to alter the course of acute lung injury in animal models. In the early phases, pulmonary hypertension was reduced, ventilation ($\dot{V}$) perfusion ($\dot{Q}$) mismatch diminished and neutrophil adherence and activation decreased. The incidence of pulmonary oedema was also less in treated subjects.

### Prostaglandin

Prostaglandins (PG) $E_1$ and $E_2$, by preventing platelet adherence, reducing pulmonary hypertension, decreasing lymphokine production,

decreasing the generation of ROS by macrophages and inducing T lymphocyte suppressor function, have been thought to be of potential therapeutic benefit. An increased 30-day survival was shown in patients with ARDS, although most were patients from a surgical ICU with inadequate documentation of pulmonary artery occlusion pressures, and a subsequent multi-centre trial of $PGE_1$ therapy failed to show a reduction in mortality.

### Antioxidants

In early ARDS or those at high risk of developing the syndrome, protection against ROS-mediated injury using N-acetyl cysteine has been shown to reduce injury. The liver frees cysteine, itself a free radical scavenger, for incorporation into glutathione, a powerful scavenger of reactive oxygen species. Following preliminary studies, a multi-centre trial is now under way. The use of specific antioxidants in ARDS is complicated by the pro-oxidant effect of many of these compounds. Lower levels of the antioxidant vitamin E have been demonstrated in patients who developed ARDS compared with those who do not, but high levels of both vitamins E and C have been shown to promote lipid peroxidation, suggesting they induce free radical-mediated damage. In the isolated perfused rat lung model, reactive oxygen scavenging with dimethylthiourea (DMTU) prevents damage caused by activated neutrophils.

### Neutrophil-endothelial cell interaction

Pentoxifylline is a methylxanthine derivative that reduces the production of TNF and IL-1 and decreases the response of neutrophils and the pulmonary endothelium to these cytokines. It also improves red cell deformability and decreases red-cell and platelet aggregation. The haemodynamic changes associated with sepsis are ameliorated, as are indices of lung injury when pentoxifylline is used either before or soon after a pulmonary insult. Oxygen delivery is maintained in models of haemodynamic shock, possibly by preventing white-cell adherence in the pulmonary and systemic microcirculations. This suggests a potential role for pentoxifylline in ARDS, although this is yet to be defined.

### Surfactant

The increased ROS-mediated activity associated with ARDS reduces the concentration of alveolar surfactant. Surfactant production by Type II pneumocytes is further influenced by hypoxia, hyperoxia and infection. Bronchiolar lavage in patients with ARDS demonstrates low levels of surfactant. In the infantile respiratory distress syndrome, instillation of surfactant has a profoundly beneficial effect on outcome. Similarly, in animal studies exogenous surfactant replacement has been shown to reduce shear forces in damaged lung and reduce injury. Trials are under way to assess to use of surfactant in ARDS.

### Manipulation of the L-arginine pathway

There is now good evidence that induction of nitric oxide (NO) synthase by inflammatory mediators contributes to the resistant hypotension of septic shock. NO is now thought to be the major component of the endothelial-derived relaxant factor. Reports of two such patients being successfully treated with an inhibitor of NO synthesis have been published this year. Conversely, the characteristic pulmonary circulatory changes of sepsis and ARDS are loss of hypoxic pulmonary vasoconstriction (HPV) and hypertension. Studies in rats have implicated NO in the modulation of HPV and have suggested that low dose TNF inhibits the action of NO prior to disrupting the endothelium. Hence, inhaled NO (20 ppm) has been used in certain centres to decrease pulmonary vascular resistance and to improve oxygenation by decreasing intravascular shunt. Results have yet to be published. Concern about the toxicity of inhaled NO has been allayed by recent experience in animals and patients. Furthermore, in many respects inhaled NO is an ideal pulmonary vasodilator as it is inactivated by haemoglobin in the circulation rapidly enough to prevent systemic actions and only dilates vessels supplying ventilated units.

## Management summary: ARDS

As soon as the diagnosis of ARDS is made, the patient must be moved to an intensive care unit where the staff are used to dealing with such cases. In patients with the established syndrome, the patient should be sedated, paralysed and intubated and full mechanical ventilatory support instigated. A balloon-tipped, flow-directed, pulmonary artery catheter of the thermodilution type should be inserted and baseline measurements of oxygen delivery and uptake made, and pulmonary and systemic vascular resistances calculated. When compared to conventional IPPV without PEEP in patients with ARDS, an I:E ratio of 4:1 has been shown to increase end expiratory lung volume and improve arterial oxygenation impressively by decreasing shunt fraction. However, this occurred at the expense of a decrease in overall oxygen delivery due to an associated fall in cardiac output. More recently, two retrospective studies have reviewed the progress of a total of 43 patients with ARDS deemed to have failed to respond to conventional ventilation and subsequently switched to PC-IRV. Each reported a significant fall in PIP and PEEP levels in association with a slight elevation in Paw. Cardiovascular performance was not compromised in patients successfully transferred to PC-IRV although the majority were managed on I:E ratios of 2:1 or 3:1. The improved gas exchange seen with IRV is thought due to more efficient alveolar recruitment and stabilisation with a secondary advancement in lung compliance and ventilatory efficiency. These changes are not immediate and some hours of therapy (with close monitoring) are required for these benefits to accrue. Although PC-IRV has not been shown to improve outcome, controlled prospective trials are in progress; until the results are available this seems to represent the optimal means of increasing arterial oxygenation whilst minimising the threat of barotrauma and the adverse haemodynamic results of PEEP.

Monoclonal antibody technology has developed to a level where binding individual mediators or receptors is now being applied to clinical practice. Such therapies will be expensive and should be introduced only after their efficacy has been proved in large well-designed trials. Costs can also be off-set against the benefits of decreased mortality in what are frequently young patients expected to recover fully, and reduced time within the intensive care unit. Thus, anti-endotoxin antibody (HA-1A, centoxin) and anti-TNF antibodies will almost certainly be reserved for patients with ARDS in association with the sepsis syndrome. The use of surfactant may be restricted to those patients in single (respiratory) organ system failure; the results of a multi centre trial are awaited. Other therapeutic interventions that will almost certainly be available within the next few years will also almost certainly be targeted towards specific sub-groups.

The discovery of an ever-increasing number of inflammatory mediators has provided new targets for immune therapy, but has also revealed a complex system with enormous redundancy, implying that a single agent is unlikely to be able to halt the process once initiated. In this respect, targeting 'initiators' or early mediators such as endotoxin is an attractive option, but depends on initiating therapy immediately after the insult which is not always feasible in the clinical setting.

Optimism about anti-inflammatory treatments has been dampened by the consistent failure of trials using corticosteroids to justify their routine use in patients with ARDS, although certain subgroups may benefit. Given the high incidence of infection complicating ARDS, immunosuppressant therapy must be used with caution. Of the new agents outlined above, inhaled NO is particularly exciting though its emerging role as an immunomodulator and its interaction with ROS remains to be characterised.

FURTHER READING

Dinh Xuan A T, Higenbottom T W, Scott J P, Wallwork J 1990 Primary pulmonary hypertension; diagnosis, medical and surgical management. Respiratory Medicine 84: 189–198

Editorial 1992. Thrombolysis for pulmonary embolus. Lancet 340: 21–22

Gray H H, Firoozan S 1992 Management of pulmonary embolus. Thorax (in press)

Griffiths M J D, Evans T W 1991 Pharmacology of shock. In: Mechanism of action of drugs in anaesthesia. Edward Arnold, London (in press)

Macnaughton P, Evans T W 1991 Adult respiratory distress syndrome. In: Recent advances in pulmonary medicine. Churchill Livingstone, Edinburgh p 1–25

Macnaughton P, Evans T W 1992 Adult respiratory distress syndrome. Lancet 339: 469–472

Madden B, Radley-Smith R, Hodson M, Khaghani A, Yacoub M 1992 Medium term results of heart and lung transplantation. Journal of Heart and Lung Transplantation (in press)

Messent M, Evans T W 1991 Adult respiratory distress syndrome. In: Progress in respiratory medicine. Butterworths Press, London (in press)

Morgan J M, McCormack D G, Griffiths M J D, Morgan C J, Barnes P J, Evans T W 1991 Adenosine as a selective pulmonary vasodilator. Circulation 84: 1145–1149

CHAPTER CONTENTS

**Cough 153**
Introduction 153
Physiology of cough 153
Causes of cough 154
Management of persistent cough 156
Drugs used to treat cough 157
   Narcotic antitussives 157
   Non-narcotic antitussive agents 158
   Expectorant drugs and mucolytics 158

**Breathlessness 159**
Physiological basis for breathlessness 159
Clinical considerations 159
Treatment 160
   Primary disease 160
   Symptomatic treatment 160
   Reducing the sensation of breathlessness 160

# 9

# Treatment of cough and breathlessness

## COUGH

### Introduction

Cough is one of the commonest symptoms of lung disease and is a frequent problem in general practice. This symptom occurs at all ages and is usually caused by upper respiratory tract infections and by cigarettee smoking. Cigarette smokers may accept cough and sputum production as 'normal' until the pattern of the cough worsens such that it interferes with social activities or causes discomfort. As with any symptom, cough has to be investigated so that a proper approach to the treatment of the underlying disease can be given. However, symptomatic treatment of cough is often necessary when it is irritating and distressing. There is a large demand for the symptomatic relief of cough as evidenced by the availability and popularity of over 90 different preparations which can be bought over the counter in the UK.

### Physiology of cough

The cough reflex represents a protective and defensive mechanism which can be under voluntary or involuntary control for the removal of mucus and any foreign particles from the larynx, trachea and larger bronchi. This reflex involves the stimulation of airway sensory nerves with vagal afferents to the cough centre in the brain stem, and the activation of motor nerves to the diaphragm, the abdominal and intercostal muscles, and the larynx. Cough receptors, which respond mainly to mechanical stimulation and deformation of the airway epithelium such as particulate matter and mucus, are localised preferentially in the trachea and carina. Other receptors, such as bronchial or pulmonary C-fibres, are preferentially stimulated by chemical stimuli such as irritant gases with a distribution throughout the tracheobronchial tree. It has been suggested that irritation of the bronchial mucosa does not lead directly to the stimulation of cough receptors, but first causes bronchoconstriction, which in turn stimulates cough receptors. However, it is now clear that cough and bronchoconstriction can be separated pharmacologically and that these two airway reflexes may have separate neural pathways. The cough reflex may be enhanced in patients with chronic persistent cough.

Cough is usually preceded by a deep inspiration followed by a rapid contraction of the expiratory muscles and closure of the glottis. Intrathoracic pressure rises with compression of gas in the trachea and airways of up to a pressure of 30 cm of mercury. The glottis then opens suddenly, leading to an explosion of air which can approach the velocity of sound. This forceful cough helps to expel mucus and foreign bodies from the major airways. Many stimuli which can cause coughing can also increase airway secretions which provide a vehicle for removing particulate matter.

## Causes of cough

Table 9.1 indicates the wide range of disease processes which may present with cough. In order to diagnose the cause of cough one must take into consideration the history, physical examination and other tests including chest radiograph, pulmonary function tests and sometimes fibreoptic bronchoscopy. In many cases, a confident diagnosis may be reached from a careful history and examination alone.

*Cigarette smoking* is an important cause of chronic cough which can disappear within a

| Table 9.1 Common causes of cough |
| --- |
| **Acute infections** |
| Tracheobronchitis |
| Bronchopneumonia |
| Viral pneumonia |
| Acute-on-chronic bronchitis |
| **Chronic infections** |
| Bronchiectasis |
| Tuberculosis |
| Cystic fibrosis |
| **Airway diseases** |
| Asthma |
| Chronic bronchitis |
| Chronic post-nasal drip |
| **Parenchymal disease** |
| Interstitial fibrosis |
| Emphysema |
| **Tumours** |
| Bronchogenic carcinoma |
| Alveolar cell carcinoma |
| Benign airway tumours |
| Mediastinal tumours |
| **Foreign body** |
| **Cardiovascular** |
| Left ventricular failure |
| Pulmonary infarction |
| Aortic aneurysm |
| **Other disease** |
| Reflux oesophagitis |
| Recurrent aspiration |
| **Drugs** |
| Angiotensin-converting enzyme inhibitors |

few weeks of cessation of smoking. Mucoid sputum production in a smoker usually indicates *chronic bronchitis*, but the expectoration of a dark yellow or green sputum may signify a bronchopulmonary infection such as in *acute bronchitis*, *bronchiectasis* or *pneumonia* and may occur frequently in patients with *cystic fibrosis*. *Upper respiratory virus infections* are probably the

---

**Box 9.1 Proposed treatments for cough**

| Treat specific underlying cause | | Symptomatic approach | |
|---|---|---|---|
| Asthma | Bronchodilators & inhaled corticosteroids | Acute cough likely to be transient, e.g. viral rhinitis | Simple linctus |
| Allergic rhinitis & post-nasal drip | Topical nasal steroids + antihistamines | Persistent cough particularly nocturnal | Opiates (codeine or pholcodeine) |
| Oesophageal reflux | H$_2$-histamine antagonist or proton pump inhibitor | Persistent intractable cough due to incurable terminal disease | Opiates (morphine or diamorphine) Local anaesthetics |
| Angiotensin-converting enzyme inhibitor | Alternative therapy | | |
| Bronchiectasis | Postural drainage. Treat infective exacerbation or airways obstruction | Cough in children | Simple linctus (paediatric) |
| Infective tracheobronchitis | Appropriate antibiotic therapy if indicated | | |

---

commonest cause of a transient self-limited cough, particularly in children, although such a cough may persist for many months. A more persistent cough, usually during the night or in the early morning, which may be associated with bronchial hyperresponsiveness (an exaggerated response of the airways to inhaled stimuli) and wheezing, should be recognised as *bronchial asthma*.

Post-nasal drip which usually presents with complaints of feeling phlegm or a drip at the back of the throat is often associated with a cough and is usually due to *nasal or sinus disease*, often allergic in origin. The presence of *allergic rhinitis* and *nasal polyps* may lead to repeated throat irritation and cough. Reflux oesophagitis with a *hiatus hernia* is now increasingly being recognised as a cause of chronic persistent cough and may only be diagnosed by therapeutic trial of specific medication, e.g. with a H$_2$-histamine antagonist or with an inhibitor of the proton pump. *Recurrent aspiration* may also present with nocturnal coughing. Patients with *congestive cardiac failure* may also complain of a chronic cough. Approximately 10% of patients on angiotensin-converting enzyme inhibitors

(e.g. captopril and enalapril) used as treatment for hypertension may develop a chronic cough not usually associated with wheezing.

Physical examination may reveal the specific cause of coughing such as signs of obstructive or restrictive lung disease, congestive cardiac failure, pleural effusions or pulmonary collapse. The chest radiograph may confirm these findings, or reveal in addition bronchiectasis, pulmonary infiltrates or emphysema. Radiographic analysis of the paranasal sinuses is helpful in patients who have a cough associated with a post-nasal drip. Pulmonary function tests may confirm obstructive or restrictive lung disease. The diagnosis of asthma underlying a resistant nocturnal cough may be supported by significant nocturnal or early morning fall in peak expiratory flow rates and by the presence of bronchial hyperresponsiveness. A fibreoptic bronchoscopy examination should be carried out if no definite cause has been found from other investigations. Computed tomography of the lungs may also be useful to diagnose or define any disease process that may underlie cough such as bronchiectasis or parenchymal disorders.

## Management of persistent cough
(Box 9.1)

The most important point about the management of cough is to look for the cause and then treat it. Thus, treatment of oesophageal reflux with an $H_2$-histamine receptor antagonist (e.g. cimetidine or ranitidine) or a proton pump inhibitor (e.g. omeprazole), and of a post-nasal drip in a patient with allergic sinorhinitis with a topical nasal steroid preparation or an $H_1$-histamine receptor antagonist (e.g. terfenadine) may be all that is needed. Patients with cough associated with therapy with angiotensin-converting should use alternative therapy.

Persistent cough may be treated symptomatically when the cause cannot be found or when satisfactory treatment of the cause is not possible. Cough becomes a troublesome symptom when it serves no useful function and causes discomfort, loss of sleep or social embarrassment. In addition, persistent cough may sometimes lead to complications such as cough fractures or syncopal episodes. It would be entirely appropriate to suppress an irritable nocturnal cough of a patient with an infective tracheobronchitis and also the cough of a patient with terminal bronchial carcinoma. The duration of symptomatic treatment would be different in the two cases. However, it is not advisable to use cough suppressants in a patient with chronic obstructive airways disease in whom cough serves the useful purpose of expelling excessive airway secretions. Advice about stopping smoking and bronchodilators would be more appropriate.

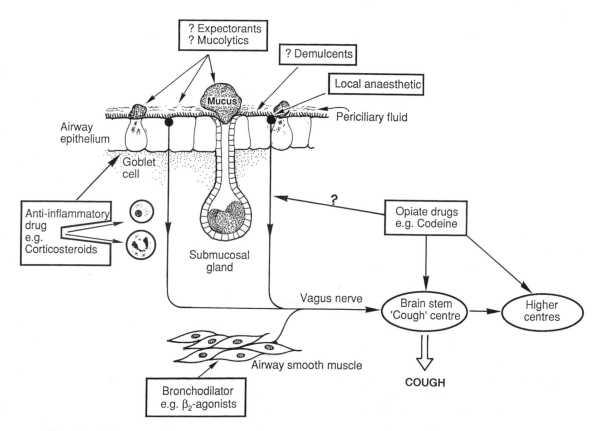

**Fig. 9.1**  Afferent pathways of the cough reflex and potential sites of action of antitussive agents.

| Table 9.2 Dose schedules of antitussive drugs | |
| --- | --- |
| Simple linctus BP | Adults 5 ml 3–4 times per day |
| Simple linctus Paediatric BP | Children 5–10 ml 3–4 times per day |
| Codeine | Adults 30–60 mg every 4–6 hours Children 1.5–2.5 mg/kg/24 hours in 4–6 doses |
| Dihydrocodeine | Adults 30 mg every 4–6 hours Children 0.5–1 mg/kg/24 hours in 4–6 doses |
| Pholcodeine | Adults 5–20 mg every 4 hours Children 2–4 mg every 6 hours |
| Dextromethorphan | Adults 15–30 mg every 4–6 hours Children 1 mg/kg/24 hours over 3–4 doses |

## Drugs used to treat cough (Table 9.2)

Drugs which can affect the complex mechanism of the cough reflex may act in several ways. They may act by inhibition of central mechanisms within the midbrain, although these mechanisms are unclear, or by reducing the response of cough receptors in the airways (Fig. 9.1).

*Opiates.* These are the most studied of all antitussive agents and although they may act by a direct action on the medullary cough centre, they may also act on sensory nerve endings which initiate cough. Details of the opiates are given below.

*Demulcents.* These form an important component of many proprietary cough preparations and many patients have the impression that they relieve dry irritating cough. Simple linctus is a demulcent with no particular pharmacological action, and contains a syrup which probably acts by lining the mucus surface with a protective layer.

*Local anaesthetics.* These are delivered locally by aerosol to the airways. They inhibit sensory neural activity and are effective antitussive agents, but also remove reflexes that protect the lung from noxious agents and should be reserved for patients with intractable cough. Their effects are transient and they should be avoided in patients with asthma or a past history of asthma because they can induce severe bronchoconstriction.

Although cough and bronchoconstriction can be separated pharmacologically, *bronchodilators* such as inhaled $\beta_2$-agonists may be effective in inhibiting cough accompanying obstructive airway disorders such as asthma and chronic bronchitis and also following fibreoptic bronchoscopy. $\beta_2$-agonists may be effective by reducing the sensitivity of cough receptors. Inhaled *corticosteroid* therapy will be effective in controlling cough associated with asthma or airway hyperresponsiveness.

### Narcotic antitussive agents

The most effective antitussive agents are the narcotic drugs such as morphine, diamorphine, codeine and the semi-synthetic derivatives which are also potent analgesics. Unfortunately at their effective doses, they also cause physical dependence, respiratory depression and gastrointestinal colic. Morphine and diamorphine are very addictive but are useful in treating uncomfortable cough or pain in patients with malignant disease of the airways and lungs. Other less addictive opiates such as codeine, dihydrocodeine and pholcodeine may be used in non-terminal illnesses. Non-narcotic antitussive agents have also been developed, but their effectiveness is not clear.

*Codeine, dihydrocodeine and pholcodeine.* Codeine is the methylether of morphine and has long been the standard centrally-acting antitussive drug against which the pharmacological and clinical effects of newer drugs have been measured. Codeine is probably still the most commonly prescribed antitussive. It has good analgesic and antitussive activity when given orally. Codeine should be used cautiously in patients with reduced hepatic function, but it can be used without dose modification in patients with renal failure. Drowsiness may be an incapacitating side-effect, together with nausea and vomiting and constipation; rarely allergic cutaneous reactions (e.g. erythema multiforme) have been described. Codeine may cause physical dependence, but this is a much smaller problem than with morphine.

Dihydrocodeine has no particular advantage over codeine and may cause more addiction than codeine. Pholcodeine is also as effective as codeine but has little or no analgesic effect. There seems little to choose between pholcodeine and codeine. Side-effects from pholcodeine are uncommon but nausea, constipation and drowsiness sometimes occur.

*Morphine, diamorphine and methadone.* These drugs should only be used for severe distressing cough which cannot be relieved by other less potent antitussives, and are therefore usually confined to patients with terminal illness such as bronchial carcinoma. In addition to their antitussive effect, these opioids also relieve pain and anxiety. They cause sedation, respiratory depression and constipation. Opioids can exacerbate wheezing through the release of histamine, but this is a rare side-effect. Diamorphine may be preferred to morphine because of its lower incidence of nausea and vomiting. Morphine may be given by mouth every 4 hours, and also by suppository. Diamorphine is preferably given by injection.

### Non-narcotic antitussives

Several non-narcotic agents have been reported to have antitussive properties but in many cases their effectiveness is not proven by properly conducted clinical trials. The most important non-narcotic antitussive is *dextromethorphan* which is a synthetic derivative of morphine with no analgesic or sedative properties. It is as effective as codeine in suppressing cough when given orally. It is commonly used as a constituent of many compound cough preparations which are sold over the counter. Side-effects are

few with the usual dose, but at higher doses dizziness, nausea and vomiting and headaches may occur. It should be avoided or used with care in patients with hepatic insufficiency as it undergoes metabolic degradation in the liver. Dextromethorphan should be used with caution also in patients on monoamine-oxidase inhibitors as cases of central nervous depression and death have occurred.

Other non-narcotic agents are of doubtful value as antitussive agents and are usually included in proprietary cough mixtures. *Noscapine* is a non-addictive, non-narcotic alkaloid from benzylisoquinolone fraction of opium. *Levopropoxyphene* is the laevo-isomer of the analgesic propoxyphene but has no analgesic properties.

*Benzonatate, caraniphen* and *carbetapentane* have local-anaesthetic and atropine-like effects but have no proven effectiveness as antitussive agents. *Antihistamines* are included in several cough mixtures but are of doubtful value, except for controlling rhinitis and post-nasal drip. Compound cough preparations should be avoided because many contain a large number of ingredients, usually in subtherapeutic doses. They also often consist of agents with opposing effects.

### Expectorant drugs and mucolytics

Various cough mixtures contain agents such as ammonium chloride and mucolytics which are thought to act as expectorants by modifying the composition of the airway surface liquid and of the sputum. Mucolytic agents such as acetylcysteine, carbocisteine, bromhexine and methylcysteine are thought to facilitate expectoration by reducing sputum viscosity in patients with chronic bronchitis. They may also prevent lung damage such as that induced by cigarette smoke by an antioxidant effect, but this effect has not been proven. A small reduction in exacerbation of bronchitis has been reported with oral acetylcysteine (200 mg twice daily), accompanied by some improvement in cough, a decrease in volume of sputum and some ease of expectoration.

However, these are not clinically important effects.

## BREATHLESSNESS

Breathlessness, dyspnoea or shortness of breath is one of the commonest symptoms felt by patients with cardiac or pulmonary disease, and the mechanisms by which these sensations are produced remain obscure. The symptom of breathlessness or dyspnoea usually encompasses a distressing sensation of laboured breathing or air hunger, which is brought on by even mild exertion in patients with cardiac or pulmonary disease. This sensation of breathlessness is distinguished from the unpleasant, but not distressing, sensation felt by healthy subjects during exercise.

## Physiological basis for breathlessness

The respiratory centre receives a number of inputs which may interact in a complex fashion to increase respiratory drive and the sensation of breathlessness. Hypoxaemia and hypercapnia can increase respiratory drive and the stimulation of airway and lung receptors such as pulmonary stretch or type J receptors may mediate dyspnoea in conditions associated with alveolar and pulmonary vascular disease. Afferent impulses are transmitted by the vagus nerves which are thought to play a major role in the perception of breathlessness. Bilateral vagal blockage with local anaesthesia has been shown to relieve the sensation of breathlessness in some patients. Other proposed mechanisms for dyspnoea are fatigue of respiratory muscles, inappropriate length–tension relationships in respiratory muscle spindles, mismatch between demand for breathing and the effort needed to achieve ventilatory needs. However, there is still no certainty as to the exact mechanisms that give rise to a sensation of breathlessness in patients with chronic cardiopulmonary disease.

---

> **Box 9.2   Causes of breathlessness**
>
> - Respiratory disease
>     - e.g.   emphysema
>             pulmonary fibrosis
>             lung collapse
>
> - Cardiovascular disease
>     - e.g.   pulmonary oedema
>             pulmonary embolism
>
> - Neuromuscular disease
>
> - Metabolic acidosis
>
> - Severe anaemia
>
> - Psychogenic

A rational approach to the pharmacological control of incapacitating breathlessness has not been possible. Some attempts have been made to distinguish the effects of drugs on the sensation of breathlessness from that on the ventilatory drive to breathe on the assumption that drugs which depress the former but not the latter will be most beneficial to patients.

## Clinical considerations

The differential diagnosis of breathlessness includes lung diseases such as chronic obstructive lung disease, asthma, pulmonary fibrosis, congestive heart failure, neuromuscular diseases and severe anaemia (Box 9.2). A careful history and physical examination are therefore basic requirements for diagnosing the cause of breathlessness. The degree of breathlessness may be assessed by determining what specific daily activity induces dyspnoea and how much the symptom interferes with lifestyle. Pulmonary function tests should be performed together with exercise testing which may help to distinguish underlying pulmonary causes from non-pulmonary causes.

In general, the sensation of dyspnoea is more intense in more advanced pulmonary disease, although some patients may experience significant dyspnoea with a relatively small impairment in lung function.

# Treatment

## Primary disease

Relief of breathlessness is most effectively achieved by treatment aimed at the primary disease. In chronic airways obstruction and asthma, specific attention should be aimed at relieving airways obstruction with $\beta_2$-agonists, anticholinergic agents and corticosteroids (Ch. 2).

## Symptomatic treatment

In some patients, the lung disease cannot be reversed such as in advanced chronic airways obstruction with emphysema or in end-stage lung fibrosis or damage and dyspnoea is a major incapacitating symptom. Long-term oxygen treatment may be helpful (Ch. 3). Therefore, measures aimed at suppressing the sensation of breathlessness are a worthwhile symptomatic goal. In addition, improving nutrition and rehabilitative exercise programmes may also improve dyspnoea. Because dyspnoea is made worse by psychological factors, psychotherapy may be of help and any psychiatric disorder should be specifically treated.

## Reducing the sensation of breathlessness

*Morphine* has been used for a long time to relieve the distress and breathlessness accompanying left ventricular failure. It has also been used in severe chronic obstructive airway disease without hypercapnia ('pink puffers') with improvement in the sensation of dyspnoea. *Dihydrocodeine* can also be effective in pink puffers and appears to affect dyspnoea more than ventilation without altering arterial carbon dioxide levels. Dihydrocodeine may cause less depression of the respiratory centre than morphine. The beneficial effect of *diazepam* at high doses of 25 mg/day in pink puffers has not been confirmed in later studies. Promethazine, a histamine $H_1$ antagonist, and chlorpromazine have also been reported to have a beneficial effect. Despite these studies, the use of drugs to control incapacitating breathlessness in chronic pulmonary disease remains unclear. The side-effects from centrally-active drugs may be substantial, in particular significant $CO_2$ retention, and the benefits may only be marginal. However, it may be worth tryingdihydrocodeine at a dose of 15–30 mg up to 3–4 times per day, being careful to monitor the patient for carbon dioxide retention. Other agents such as diazepam, promethazine or chlorpromazine may be tried. It must be remembered that these drugs may by themselves cause a restriction in daily activities by causing severe drowsiness.

FURTHER READING

Campbell E J M, Howell J B L 1963 The sensation of breathlessness. British Medical Bulletin 19: 36–54

Fuller R W, Jackson D M 1990 Physiology and treatment of cough. Thorax 45: 425–430

Irwin R S, Curley F J, French C L 1990 Chronic cough: the spectrum and frequency of causes. Key components of the diagnostic evaluation, and outcome of specific therapy. American Review of Respiratory Disease 141: 640–647

Karlsson J-A, Sant'Ambrogio G, Widdicombe J 1988 Afferent neural pathways in cough and reflex bronchoconstriction. Journal of Applied Physiology 65: 1007–1023

Stark R D 1988 Dyspnoea: assessment and pharmacological manipulation. European Respiratory Journal 1988 1: 280–287

CHAPTER CONTENTS

**Introduction 161**

**Drug-related bronchospasm and cough 162**
ß-adrenergic blockers 162
Aspirin sensitivity 162
Inhibitors of angiotensin-converting enzyme 163
Agents administered by inhalation 163
  Aerosolised medications for asthma 163
  Aerosolised pentamidine 163

**Drug-induced pulmonary injury 163**
Drugs used as chemotherapeutic agents 164
Drugs used for inflammatory arthritis 164
Cardiovascular drugs 164

**Drug-induced pulmonary eosinophilia 165**

**Drug-induced pulmonary oedema 165**

# 10

# Drug-induced pulmonary disease

## INTRODUCTION

The list of drugs implicated in causing side-effects to the lungs is growing rapidly and respiratory symptoms are a common manifestation of adverse drug reactions. Over the last 20 years, the number of commonly used agents capable of toxic damage to the lungs has more than doubled. It is difficult to obtain an exact incidence of serious pulmonary side-effects induced by individual drugs. Many reactions appear to be idiosyncratic and sporadic and a specific diagnosis of drug-induced lung disease is often difficult to ascertain because of lack of typical features and because the underlying disease may also affect the lungs. However, it appears that drug-induced pulmonary complications only occur in a small proportion of the population who receive therapeutic drugs. Nevertheless, the diagnosis of drug-induced pulmonary disease should remain a challenge for the physician and with the introduction of many new drugs, it is important to keep up-to-date with drugs that may induce pulmonary side-effects. The clinician should keep a high index of suspicion that any drug may potentially affect the lung and that most of the pulmonary reactions are reversible if the drug is stopped in time. Drugs may cause pulmonary parenchymal disease, as well as disease of the airways.

## DRUG-RELATED BRONCHOSPASM AND COUGH (Box 10.1)

### $\beta$-adrenergic blockers

$\beta$-blockers are used widely in the treatment of ischaemic heart disease and hypertension and can induce bronchospasm in patients with asthma. Therefore, $\beta$-blockers should be avoided in asthma, and also in patients with chronic obstructive airways disease, in case they have unrecognised asthma. Bronchoconstriction caused by $\beta$-blockers appears to be mediated by inhibition of the $\beta_2$-receptor subclass. Cardioselective $\beta$-blockers for the $\beta_1$-receptor subclass such as metoprolol and atenolol have been developed, and some may also possess intrinsic sympathomimetic activity, such as acebutolol and pindolol. These can be used with a relative degree of safety in patients with obstructive lung disease if there are compelling clinical reasons. However, the utmost care must be taken particularly in asthmatics with very hyperreactive airways and when these $\beta$-blockers are used at high doses.

Bronchospasm can also develop in asthmatic patients after the use of timolol eye drops, a non-selective $\beta$-blocker used for the treatment of glaucoma. Symptoms can be quite severe, even leading to respiratory arrest, and these usually develop within a few minutes of administration. Systemic reactions to timolol eye drops result from its systemic absorption and its high potency as a nonselective $\beta$-blocker.

Bronchospasm induced by $\beta$-adrenergic blockers is probably mediated by the activation of airway cholinergic nerves and the treatment of choice for $\beta$-blocker bronchospasm is inhaled anti-cholinergic medication. Inhaled $\beta$-agonists are usually not effective. $\beta$-blocker medications should be avoided in patients with asthma and alternative treatments should be used. For example, for hypertension, calcium channel blockers and inhibitors of angiotensin-converting enzyme may be used instead.

> **Box 10.1    Drug-related bronchospasm and cough**
>
> - $\beta$-blockers
> - Aspirin
> - Non-steroidal anti-inflammatory drugs
> - Nebulised pentamidine
> - Use of metered dose inhalers

## Aspirin sensitivity

A small proportion of asthmatic subjects develop worsening of asthma with aspirin, with an incidence varying from 4 to 20% of asthmatic patients. Aspirin-sensitive asthmatics usually develop symptoms later in life; rhinitis and nasal polyposis and cross-reactivity with other non-steroidal anti-inflammatory drugs such as phenylbutazone or indomethacin is well recognised. Aspirin-induced bronchospasm usually develops in the third to fourth decade and tends to be more common in women. The pathogenesis of this condition is unclear, but one possibility is an imbalance in the production of the bronchodilating and bronchoconstricting prostaglandins or shunting of arachidonic acid metabolism toward the lipoxygenase pathway with the increased production of bronchoconstrictor leukotrienes. Recently, a leukotriene antagonist has been shown to inhibit aspirin-induced bronchoconstriction.

Clearly, aspirin and non-steroidal anti-inflammatory drugs should be avoided in aspirin-sensitive asthmatic patients. Many proprietary drugs contain acetylsalicylic acid and patients should be told to check carefully the constituent of any proprietary drugs they take. Even indomethacin eye drops have been reported to precipitate life-threatening asthmatic reactions in such patients. Paracetamol is usually tolerated in patients who require analgesia. Desensitisation may be a potentially useful approach in a minority of aspirin-sensitive patients who still require the use of such medications.

# Inhibitors of angiotensin-converting enzyme

Cough is an increasingly well recognised side-effect of all angiotensin-converting enzyme (ACE) inhibitors such as captopril and enalapril, with a reported incidence of 15% occurring more commonly in women. A dry, persistent cough may develop within a few days or even months of starting medication and usually disappears within 1–2 weeks of cessation. There have been no reports of asthma associated with cough induced by angiotensin-converting enzyme inhibitors. ACE inhibitors can be used in patients with airways obstruction. Non-steroidal anti-inflammatory drugs may inhibit ACE inhibitor induced cough.

# Agents administered by inhalation

### Aerosolised medications for asthma

Cough and bronchospasm may occur with the use of metered dose inhalers, and these effects have been attributed to inert propellants and dispersants used in these inhalers. Up to 20% of asthmatics attending an outpatient clinic have been reported to develop cough and bronchospasm on inhaling beclomethasone dipropionate aerosol, an effect attributed to the propellant and dispersant. Using a dry powder inhaler instead may overcome these problems.

Paradoxical bronchospasm has been reported with nebulised solutions of ipratropium bromide, which has been attributed variously to hypotonicity of the nebulised solution and the benzalkonium preservative. These possibilities have now been corrected and such paradoxical bronchospasm is rare. If it occurs, withdrawal of the drug from the patients is warranted.

### Aerosolised pentamidine

Aerosolised pentamidine, used for prophylaxis and treatment of *Pneumocystis curinii*, frequently induced cough and bronchospasm particularly in patients with hyperreactive airways. Pre-

treatment with inhaled bronchodilators such as $\beta_2$-agonists usually prevents these symptoms.

# DRUG-INDUCED PULMONARY INJURY (Box 10.2)

A large number of drugs can adversely affect the lung parenchymal tissues, possibly by different mechanisms, and it is therefore important for the clinician to be aware of the ability of certain drugs to cause pulmonary injury. Some of

---

**Box 10.2    Drugs that may cause parenchymal pulmonary disease**

CHEMOTHERAPEUTIC AGENTS
Azathioprine
Bleomycin
Busulphan
Carmustine (BCNU)
Cyclophosphamide
Cytosine arabinoside
Etoposide (VP-16)
Melphalan
Methotrexate
Nitrosureas
Procarbazine
Vinblastine

ANTIBIOTICS
Amphotericin B
Nitrofurantoin
Sulphasalazine
Sulphonamides
Pentamidine

ANTI-INFLAMMATORY/IMMUNOSUPPRESSIVE AGENTS
Cyclosporin
Gold
Methotrexate
Penicillamine

CARDIOVASCULAR DRUGS
Amiodarone
Tocainide
Fibrinolytic agents

OTHER MISCELLANEOUS AGENTS
Oxygen
Methysergide
Radiation
Hydrochlorothiazide

the mechanisms that may be involved in pulmonary injury caused by drugs include:

- a direct cytotoxic effect on the alveolar-capillary endothelium by agents such as cytotoxic drugs;
- production of oxygen radicals to cause oxidant injury, as by nitrofurantoin;
- immune-induced injury as may occur during drug-induced systemic lupus erythematosus.

In addition, some agents with immunosuppressive properties such as methotrexate or cyclosporin may predispose patients to opportunistic pulmonary infections, (e.g. *Pneumocystis carinii* pneumonia). However, other currently unknown mechanisms may also operate.

## Drugs used as chemotherapeutic agents

Pulmonary disease induced by chemotherapeutic agents such as bleomycin, methotrexate and cyclophosphamide have become a major problem over the last 10 years. Carmustine (BCNU)-induced pulmonary fibrosis may occur many years after chemotherapy. Pulmonary disease induced by these agents must be differentiated from other pulmonary conditions which these patients may also present with, such as opportunistic infection as well as recurrence of the lung disease for which the patient is being treated. However, in most cases, the diagnosis remains one of exclusion, although appropriate histological studies may eliminate the other possibilities. The clinical presentation may vary according to the chemotherapeutic agent, varying from an acute picture to that of a more slow, chronic onset of dyspnoea, non-productive cough and sometimes fever. Auscultation of the lungs may reveal fine inspiratory crackles and the chest radiograph may show a diffuse interstitial pattern.

## Drugs used for inflammatory arthritis

Sodium aurothiomalate (gold salts) used for the treatment of rheumatoid arthritis may cause a diffuse interstitial fibrosis. Symptoms of breathlessness with or without fever may develop slowly over weeks or months after start of weekly injections of sodium aurothiomalate. Gold-induced pneumonitis is distinct from lung fibrosis induced by rheumatoid arthritis in that it improves spontaneously on stopping gold injections or regresses with the use of corticosteroids. Methotrexate has been reported to cause a granulomatous pneumonitis, which usually responds to discontinuation of the drug and administration of high-dose prednisone.

Penicillamine which is also used for treatment of rheumatoid arthritis may affect the lung through the induction of systemic lupus erythematosus, with the production of pleural effusion and sometimes of an alveolitis. Broncholitis obliterans with organising pneumonia has also been described with drugs used for the treatment of rheumatoid arthritis such as gold salts and penicillamine. This condition has also been associated with treatment with bleomycin and amiodarone.

## Cardiovascular drugs

Amiodarone is an antiarrhythmic agent which has been associated with a number of side-effects including corneal microdeposits, peripheral neuropathy, liver abnormalities, and dysfunction of the thyroid including hypothyroidism and hyperthyroidism. The most serious side-effect, however, is an interstitial pneumonitis which occurs in up to 6% of patients and may be fatal. Although the mechanism of its pulmonary toxicity is unknown, it induces a distinctive histology consisting of foamy alveolar macrophages containing lamellar inclusions. Symptoms of amiodarone-pulmonary toxicity may include breathlessness, non-productive cough and a low-grade fever. A diffuse interstitial or alveolar process may be seen on the chest radiograph and increased lung density of pulmonary opacities due to the deposition of amiodarone can be seen on computed tomographic examination of the lungs. Withdrawal of amiodarone usually produces significant improvement, with further beneficial effect of oral corticosteroids given over a period of months.

Hydralazine and procainamide can induce systemic lupus erythematosus with a large element of pleuropulmonary involvement. Tocainide, an antiarrhythmic agent, may induce interstitial alveolitis with fibrosis within a few weeks of administration.

## DRUG-INDUCED PULMONARY EOSINOPHILIA

Many drugs induce pulmonary infiltrates associated with blood eosinophilia, including nitrofurantoin, methotrexate, salicylates, sulphonamides, penicillin and naproxen. Symptoms of breathlessness on exertion and cough usually develop within a few days of starting the drug and resolve on withdrawal of the drug.

## DRUG-INDUCED PULMONARY OEDEMA

Development of noncardiogenic pulmonary oedema has been documented with opiates (heroin, methadone and propoxyphene), intravenous $\beta_2$-adrenergic agonists (terbutaline and ritrodine used in pregnant women in the treatment of premature labour), and acetylsalicylic acid (usually in overdose).

FURTHER READING

Cooper J A D (ed) 1990 Drug-induced pulmonary disease. Clinics Chest Medicine 11: 1–190

Rosenow E C, Myers J L, Swensen S J, Pisani R J 1991 Drug-induced pulmonary disease: an update. Chest 102: 239–250

# Index

## A

Abscesses, lung, 78
Acetazolamide, 64
  in hypercarbia, 57
N-Acetylcysteine (NAC), in COPD, 54
Acquired immune deficiency
  syndrome see AIDS
Acrolein, toxicity, 119
ACTH, ectopic, lung cancer, 128
Adenosine, in primary pulmonary
  hypertension, 136
Adenosine 3, 5 monophosphate, and
  adenyl cyclase activation, 5, 18
Adenosine receptor antagonism,
  theophylline, 26-27
Adenyl cyclase
  inhibition, G-protein coupled
    receptors, 5
  stimulation
    and cAMP levels, 5, 18
    G-protein coupled receptors, 4, 5
Adrenal suppression, by
  corticosteriods, 34
Adrenaline, 16
  disadvantages, 19-20
  obstructive airway diseases, 19-20
Adriamycin (doxorubicin), lung
  cancer, 119
Adult respiratory distress syndrome
  (ARDS), 145-152
  antioxidants, 150
  and L-Arginine pathway, 151
  causes, 147-148, 149
  cytokine response modulation,
    149-150
  extracorporeal gas exchange, 147
  inflammatory mediators,
    147-148, 149
  lung pathology, 145
  management summary, 151-152

NSAIDs, 150
pharmacotherapy, new approaches,
  148-151
prostaglandins, 150
surfactant, 151
ventilation, new modes, 146-147
Affinity, drug-receptor, 7
Agonists, 7
  partial, 7
AIDS
  CMV infections, 93-94
  incidence, 85, 86
  lung infection prevention, 94-95
  mycobacterial infections, 85-95
  Pneumocystis carinii pneumonia
    (PCP), 89-93
    general measures, 92
  see also HIV infection
Airflow limitation, chronic see COAD
Airway function, corticosteroid
  effects, 32
Allergen avoidance, asthma, 38-39
Almitrine bismesylate, respiratory
  stimulation, 56
Alpha 1-antitrypsin deficiency,
  emphysema, 15
Alpha 1-protease inhibitor, COAD, 44
Alpha-methyldopa,
  DOPA mimicking, 9
Alveolitis, fibrosing, cryptogenic, 116
Amikacin, 69
Aminoglycosides, 69
  side-effects, 69
Aminophylline, 58, 63
  effects on diaphragm, 27
  intravenous, acute asthma, 41
Amiodarone, pulmonary toxicity,
  164-165
Amoxycillin, 68
  clavulanic acid combination, 68
  otitis media, 73
  sinusitis, 72
Ampicillin, 68

otitis media, 73
Analeptics, respiratory stimulation, 55
Anaphylaxis, adrenaline, 19
Angiotensin-converting enzyme
  (ACE) inhibitors
  contraindications, 45
  cough induction, 155, 163
Anorexia, treatment, in lung cancer,
  129-130
Antagonism
  competitive, 7
  functional, 7-8
Antagonists, 7
Antibiotics
  action mechanisms, 68
  in respiratory infections, 67-71
Anticholinergics
  clinical use, 24
  mode of action, 23-24
  obstructive airway disease, 23-25
  side-effects, 24-25
Anticoagulation, primary pulmonary
  hypertension, 135
Antidiuretic hormone, inappropriate
  secretion, SCLC, 127-128
Antihistamines, 37
  in cough mixtures, 158
Anti-inflammatory drugs
  COAD, 43-44
  obstructive airway diseases, 30-38
  see also Corticosteroids; NSAIDs:
    Steroids
Antioxidants, in ARDS, 150
Antituberculosis drugs, 98
  bactericidal activity, 107
  cutaneous reactions, 106
  hypersensitivity reactions,
    challenge doses, 106
  intermittent use suitability, 107-108
  and liver impairment, 100, 110
  and pregnancy, 110-111
  and renal impairment, 110
  resistance prevention, 107

sterilising action, 107
see also individual drugs
Antitussives
in COAD, 43
narcotic, 157-158
non-narcotic, 158
Apnoea
idiopathic, of prematurity, 56
see also Sleep apnoea
ARDS see Adult respiratory distress syndrome (ARDS)
L-Arginine pathway, and ARDS, 151
Arthralgia, pyrazinamide-associated, 104
Arthritis, drug therapy, and lung parenchymal disease, 164
Aspirin
cyclo-oxygenase block, 9
sensitivity in asthma, 44-45, 162
Asthma, 9, 38-42
acute
corticosteroid therapy, 35
severe, 40-42
aerosolised medications, cough/bronchospasm induction, 163
anticholinergic agents, 24
and aspirin sensitivity, 44-45, 162
brittle, 42
bronchospasm, drug-related, 162-163
chronic
auranofin therapy, 38
corticosteroid therapy, 30, 35-36
COAD differentiation, 13
deaths, and β-agonists, 21-22
definition, 13
difficult, 42, 43
eosinophilic inflammation, 15
epidemiology, 14
exacerbations, management plan, 40, 41
exercise-induced, 41
immunomodulators, 46
in infants, 42
inflammatory cells, mediators/effects, 15
lipid mediator antagonists/inhibitors, 46
low-dose methotrexate, 38
management guidelines, 38-40
morbidity, and β-agonists, 22
new drugs, 45-46
nocturnal, 41
occupational, allergen avoidance, 39
pathophysiology, 14-15
in pregnancy, 42
premenstrual, 42
steroid-resistant, 33, 42
theophylline, 27
therapy, stepwise approach, 39-40
Atropine, 23
lipophilicity, 2

Atropine methylnitrate, 23
Azithromycin, 69
Azlocillin, 68
AZT, 86, 87, 87-88
Aztreonam, 71

## B

β$_2$-agonists, inhaled, long-acting, 45
β$_2$-selective agonists, 19, 20
β$_2$-adrenergic agonists, 16-23
administration modes, 19-21
airway smooth muscle relaxation, 17-18
chemistry, 17
clinical use, 23
development from catecholamines, 16, 17
drug choice, 19-20
long-acting, 19, 20
mode of action, 17-19
safety, 21-22
side-effects, 21
tolerance, 22
β-blockers
bronchospasm induction, 162
contraindication in asthma, 44
β-receptors, corticosteroid effects, 32
Barotrauma, and ARDS therapy, 145
Beclomethasone dipropionate (BDP)
aerosol, cough/bronchospasm induction, 163
anti-asthma potency, 31
structure, 30
Benzonatate, 158
Bone marrow transplantation, autologous, 122
Breathlessness, 159-160
causes, 159
clinical aspects, 159-160
in lung cancer, treatment, 126, 129
physiology, 159
primary disease treatment, 160
sensation of, reduction, 160
short-burst oxygen therapy, 54
symptomatic treatment, 160
visual analogue scale, 53, 54
Bronchiectasis, 82
antibiotic therapy, 82
associated conditions, 82
Bronchiolitis obliterans, drug-induced, 164
Bronchitis
chronic desquamative eosinophilic, asthma, 13
see also Chronic bronchitis
Bronchoalveolar lavage, PCP diagnosis, 87
Bronchoconstriction, paradoxical, ipratropium-associated, 25, 163
Bronchodilators, 16-30

Bronchoscopy, PCP diagnosis, 87-88
Bronchospasm, drug-related, 162-163
Budesonide
anti-asthma potency, 31
structure, 30
BW566, in PCP, 91

## C

Calcitonin, in hypercalcaemia, 127
Calcium, smooth muscle, mobilisation, theophylline effects, 27
Calcium channel blockers, in primary pulmonary hypertension, 136-137
Candida albicans, 87
Capreomycin, in tuberculosis, 105
Caraniphen, 158
Carbapenems, 71
Carbenicillin, 68
Carbetapentane, 158
Carbon dioxide, extracorporeal removal, in ARDS, 147
Carbonic anhydrase inhibition, in respiratory failure, 56-57
Carboplatin, in lung cancer, 120-121
Cardiovascular drugs, lung parenchymal disease induction, 164-165
Catechol-O-methyltransferase (COMT), catecholamine metabolism, 17
Catecholamines
β-agonist development, 16, 17
endogenous
secretion, and theophylline, 27
uptake mechanisms, 17, 18
metabolism, 17
Cavernous sinus thrombosis, 72
CD4 lymphocyte count
and AZT therapy, 88-89
PCP, 89, 92
Cefotaxime, 69
Cefoxtin, 69
Cefsulodin, 69
Ceftazidime, 69
Cefuroxime, 69
sinusitis, 72
Cephalexin, 69
Cephalosporins, 69-71
nephrotoxicity, 69
Cephamandole, 69
Cetirizine, lipophilicity, 2
Chlorpromazine, 160
Chlortetracycline, 70
Cholinergic neural pathways, bronchoconstriction in asthma, 23-24
Chronic bronchitis, 82-83
and COAD, 15
corticosteroid therapy, 36
definition, 14

and upper respiratory virus infections, 83
Chronic obstructive airway disease (COAD) *see* COAD
Chronic obstructive pulmonary disease *see* COPD
Cigarette smoking
 COAD, 13, 14
 COPD, 139
 lung cancer, 116-117
 lung damage, and mucolytics, 158-159
Cilastin, 71
Ciprofloxacin, 70, 71
Cisplatin, 126
 in lung cancer, 120-121
Clarithromycin, 69
Clavulanic acid, 68
Clindamycin, 71
 primaquine combination, in PCP, 91
Cloxacillin, 68
COAD, 9
 acute exacerbations, 43
 alpha 1-protease inhibitor therapy, 44
 anti-inflammatory drugs, 43-44
 anticholinergic agents, 24, 25
 asthma differentiation, 13
 breathlessness, drug therapy, 44
 bronchodilator treatment, 43
 definition, 13
 epidemiology, 14
 inhaled steroids, 36
 management/treatment aims, 42-43
 mucolytics and antitussives, 43
 oxygen therapy, 43
 pathophysiology, 15-16
 theophylline, 29-30
Co-amoxyclav
 epiglottitis, 73
 sinusitis, 72
Codeine, 157-158
Continuous positive pressure ventilation (CPAP), oxygen therapy, 51, 52
COPD
 epidemiology, 50
 and malnutrition, 59-60
 mucociliary function, 54
 N-acetylcysteine, 54
 portable oxygen therapy, 53-54
 respiratory stimulants, 55-56
 secondary pulmonary hypertension, 132
 vasodilator therapy, 138
Cor pulmonale, 44, 49, 133, 138, 139
 epidemiology, 50
 hypoxic, 139
 respiratory failure, 57
Corticosteroids
 administration routes, 33-34
 anti-asthma potency, 31

anti-inflammatory effects, 31-32
 chemistry, 30-31
 clinical use, 35-36
 inhaled, 33-34
 pharmacokinetics, 33
 products, 34
 intravenous, 33
 local side-effects, 35
 mode of action, 31-32
 obstructive airway diseases, 30-36
 oral administration, 33
 pharmacokinetics, 32-33
 side-effects, 34-35
 systemic side-effects, 34-35
 *see also individual steroids*
Co-trimoxazole, 70, 73
 adverse reactions, 89-90
 chronic bronchitis, 83
 PCP prophylaxis, 94
 PCP therapy, 89-90
 sinusitis, 72
 versus dapsone/trimethoprim, in PCP, 91
 versus pentamidine, in PCP, 90
Cough, 153-159
 causes, 154-156
 drug therapy, 157-159
  *see also* Antitussives; Expectorants; Mucolytics
 drug-related, 155, 162-163
 persistent, management, 155, 156-157
 physiology, 153-154
 receptors, 154
 treatment, in lung cancer, 126, 129
Cromakalin, 45
*Cryptococcus neoformans*, 87
Cyclo-oxygenase inhibitors, 37-38
Cyclophosphamide
 lung cancer, 118-119
 pre-dosing effects, 119
 side-effects, 118-119
Cycloserine, in tuberculosis, 105
Cyclosporin A, in asthma, 38
Cystic fibrosis (CF)
 neutrophil elastase inhibition, 9
 recurrent respiratory infections, 81-82
  antibiotic therapy, 81-82
Cystitis, haemorrhagic, cyclophosphamide-related, 119
Cytokines
 formation inhibition, by corticosteroids, 32
 gene coding inhibition, 7
 receptors, 3
 response modulation, in ARDS, 149-150
Cytomegalovirus (CMV) infection, in AIDS, 87, 93-94
Cytotoxic agents
 lung cancer, 118-121
 lung parenchymal disease

induction, 163, 164
 side-effects, 121
 *see also individual agents*

D

Dapsone-trimethoprim combination in PCP, 90-91
 versus co-trimoxazole, in PCP, 91
Datura plants, 23
Deep venous thrombosis (DVT), 139, 140-141
 diagnosis, 140
 prevention/therapy, 140-141
Dehydration, in pneumonia, 78
Demeclocycline, 70
Desensitisation, drugs, 8
Dexamethasone, 30
Dextromethorphan, 158
Diamorphine, 158
diazepam, 44, 160
Dideoxycytidine (ddc), antiretroviral therapy, 89
Dideoxyinosine (ddI), antiretroviral therapy, 89
Digitalis, in respiratory muscle fatigue, 59
Digoxin, in respiratory muscle fatigue, 59
Dihydrocodeine, 44, 157-158
 in breathlessness, 160
Diphosphonates, in hypercalcaemia, 127
Diuretics, respiratory failure, 57
Dons CPAP mask, 51
Doxepram, respiratory stimulation, 55, 63-64
Doxycycline, 70
Drug-receptor interactions, 7-8
Drugs
 absorption, 1-2
 biotransformation, 2
 blood level, equation, 2
 clearance, 3-4
 cough/bronchospasm induction, 155, 162-163
 delivery routes, 9-11
 desensitisation, 8
 distribution, 2
 excretion routes, 3
 inhalation, 9-10
 lipophilic, central side-effects, 2
 lung parenchymal disease induction, 163-165
 oral route, 10-11
 *pKa*, 2
 potentiation, 8
 pulmonary disease induction, 160-165
 synergism, 8
 tolerance, 8

Dry powder inhalers, 10
DVT *see* Deep venous thrombosis (DVT)
Dysphagia, in lung cancer,
    radiotherapy, 126, 130
Dyspnoea *see* Breathlessness

## E

Ectopic ACTH syndrome,
    lung cancer, 128
Efficacy, drugs, 7
Eflornithine (DFMO), in PCP, 91
Electrolyte disturbance,
    in pneumonia, 78
Emphysema
    and COAD, 13
    neutrophil elastase inhibition, 9
Enprofylline, 26
Enzymes, drug interaction, 8-9
Eosinophilia, pulmonary, drug-
    induced, 195
Epiglottitis, 73
Erythromycin, 69
    pharyngitis, 73
Ethambutol
    adverse reactions, 102
    dosages, 98, 99, 102
    in tuberculosis, 102
Ethanol, lipophilicity, 2
Ethionamide, in tuberculosis, 105
Etopside, in lung cancer, 120
Expectorants, 158-159
Extracorporeal gas exchange (ECGE),
    in ARDS, 147

## F

Fenoterol
    and asthma deaths, 21, 22
    and asthma morbidity, 22
Frusemide/amiloride combination,
    respiratory failure, 57

## G

Gene transcription, regulating
    receptors, 6-7, 8
Gentamycin, 69
Glaucoma, ipratropium-associated, 25
Glucocorticoid receptors
    DNA interaction, 4
    and gene transcription, 6-7, 8
Glucocorticoid therapy, PCP, 91-92
Gold, in asthma, 38
G-protein coupled receptors, 2, 3, 5-6
G-protein receptors, phospholipase C,
    PIP2 hydrolysis, 6

G-proteins, 4-5
Growth factors, receptors, 3

## H

Haemolytic anaemia/haemolysis,
    rifampicin-related, 100
*Haemophilus influenzae*, COAD, 43
Heart-lung transplantation, in primary
    pulmonary hypertension,
    130, 137
Heparin
    deep venous thrombosis
        prevention/therapy, 140-141
    in pulmonary embolus, 142-143
Hepatitis, antituberculosis
        drug-related, 101, 106-107
Hepatotoxicity, pyrazinamide-
    associated, 103-104
High frequency jet ventilation (HFJV),
    in ARDS, 146-147
*Histoplasma capsulatum*, 87
HIV infection, 85
    antiretroviral treatment, 88-89
    pulmonary disease
        aetiological diagnosis, 86-88
        bronchoscopy, 87-88
        diagnostic tests, 86-88
        induced sputum tests, 86
        non-invasive tests, 86
        open-lung biopsy, 88
    *see also* AIDS
Hudson mask, 51
Human immunodeficiency virus (HIV)
    infection *see* HIV infection
Hydralazine, 165
Hydrocortisone, structure, 30
Hydroxyzine, lipophilicity, 2
Hypercalcaemia, and lung cancer, 127
Hypercarbia, acetazolamide, 57
Hypertension, pulmonary, 44, 131-139
    catheter studies, 134
    chest radiography, 133-134
    classification, 132
    clinical findings, 133
    diagnosis, 133-134
    electro/echocardiogram, 134
    epidemiology, 132-133
    haematology, 134
    investigations, 133-134
    primary
        diagnostic criteria, 132
        therapy, 134-137
    prognosis, 139
    pulmonary function tests (PFT), 134
    secondary, 137-138
        causes, 132, 133
    therapeutic prospects, 139
    therapy, 134-138
    tissue diagnosis, 134
Hypertrophic pulmonary

    osteoarthropathy (HPOA),
    lung cancer, 128
Hypokalaemia
    β-agonist-associated, 21
Hypoxaemia
    β-agonist-associated, 21
    in pneumonia, oxygen therapy, 78
Hypoxia, COAD, 15-16

## I

Ifosfamide, 125
Imipenem, 71
Immunoglobulin $G_2$ deficiency, AIDS, 92
Immunomodulators, in asthma, 46
Immunosuppression, and
    tuberculosis, 111
Immunosuppressive therapy,
    obstructive airway diseases, 38
Immunotherapy, obstructive airway
    diseases, 38
Indomethacin, 150
Infections, respiratory, 67
    antibiotics, 67-71
    *see also* Lower *and* Upper
        respiratory tract infections
Inferior vena cava, surgical
    interruption, pulmonary
    embolus, 143-144
Inhaled drugs, 9-10
    delivery methods, 9-10
    particle size, 9
    pharmacokinetics, 9
Interleukin-1, gene coding
    inhibition, 7
Inverse ratio ventilation (IRV)
    in ARDS, 146
    pressure-controlled (PC-IRV), 146
    volume-controlled (VC-IRV), 146
Ion channel receptors, 6
Ipratropium bromide, 23, 24
    effects on taste, 25
    lipophilicity, 2
    paradoxical bronchospasm, 41, 163
Isoniazid
    adverse reactions, 100-102
    dosages, 98, 99, 101
    fast/slow acelylators, 101
    in tuberculosis, 100-102
    tuberculosis prevention, AIDS, 94
Isoprenaline, 16-17
    obstructive airway diseases, 20

## K

Kaolin-cephalin clotting time
    (KCCT), 140
Kaposi's sarcoma, 86, 94
    bronchoscopy appearances, 88
Ketotifen, 37

# L

β-Lactams, 71
Lambert Eaton myasthenic syndrome (LEMS), 128
Laryngitis, tuberculous, 112
Laryngotracheitis, 73
Legionnaire's disease, 74
Lemakalin, 45
Leukotriene antagonists, 46
Levopropoxyphene, 158
Lipid mediator antagonists/ inhibitors, 46
Lipocortin, production by corticosteroids, 31
5-Lipoxygenase inhibitors, 46
  in asthma, 9
Liver impairment, and antituberculosis drugs, 100, 110
Lower respiratory tract infections, 73-83
  cystic fibrosis, 81-82
  recurrent, 80-83
LPS1 neutralisation, in ARDS, 149
Lung cancer, 115
  cell type/doubling times, 117
  cigarette smoking, 116-117
  cytotoxic chemotherapy, 118-121
  epidemiology, 115-117
  incidence, 115-116
    developing countries, 117
  mortality, 115, 116
  paraneoplastic syndromes, 127-128
  terminal care, 128-130
  treatment problems, 117-119
  see also Non-small cell (NSCLC); Small cell lung cancer (SCLC)

# M

Macrolides, 69-70
Malnutrition, and COPD, 59-60
Mary Catterall (MC) mask, 51
Mast cell stabilisers, 37
Mechanical ventilation, non-invasive, respiratory failure, 57
Meclofenamate, 150
Medroxyprogesterone, 56
  sleep apnoea, 64
Membrane oxygen, extracorporeal (ECMO), in ARDS, 147
Meningitis, tuberculous, drug therapy, 111
Metered dose inhalers (MDIs), 9-10
Methadone, 158
Methicillin, 68
Methotrexate, 164
  low-dose, in asthma, 38
  in lung cancer, 121
Methylxanthines, 25-30
  respiratory muscle fatigue, 58

respiratory stimulation, 55-56
Minitracheostomy, respiratory failure, 62-63
Mithramycin, in hypercalcaemia, 127
Mitomycin, C, 125
Monoamine oxidase (MAO), cate catecholamine metabolism, 17
Monoclonal antibodies, ARDS therapy, 149
Morphine, 158
  in breathlessness, 160
Mountain sickness, 57
Mucolytics, 158-159
  in COAD, 43
  in respiratory failure, 54-55
Mucus secretion, and anticholinergics, 24-25
Muscle tremor, β-agonist-associated, 21
Myasthenia gravis, streptomycin contraindication, 103
Mycobacterial infections, atypical, 109, 110, 112
Mycobacterium avium intracellulare, 112
  in AIDS, 85, 93
Mycobacterium kansasii, 112
Mycobacterium tuberculosis
  in AIDS, 85, 86, 93
  PCP co-infection, 87

# N

Nasal cannulae, oxygen therapy, 51
Nasal CPAP, sleep apnoea, 61-62, 64
Nasal intermittent positive pressure ventilation (NIPPV), 57, 60
Nebulisers, 10
Nedocromil sodium (NS), 37
Neuropathy, peripheral, isoniazid-related, 101-102
Neutrophil-endothelial cell interaction, in ARDS, 148, 149, 150-151
Nicotine, lipophilicity, 2
Nikethamide, respiratory stimulation, 55
Non-small cell lung cancer (NSCLC)
  chemotherapy, 124-125
    response rates, 124-125
  complications, palliative radiotherapy, 126-127, 129, 130
  growth rates, 117
  radiotherapy, 125-127, 129, 130
Norfloxacin, 70
Noscapine, 158
NSAIDs
  in ARDS, 150
  contraindication in asthma, 44-45, 162
Nutritional therapy, COPD, 59-60

# O

Obstructive airway diseases, 13-47
  anticholinergics, 23-25
  anti-inflammatory agents, 30-38
  β-adrenergic agonists, 16-23
  chronic see COAD
  contraindicated drugs, 44-45
  drug choice, 19-20
  eepidemiology, 14
  immunosuppressive therapy, 38
  pathophysiology, 14-16
  theophylline, 25-30
  see also individual diseases
Obstructive pulmonary disease, chronic see COAD
Oedema
  peripheral, 44
  pulmonary, drug-induced, 195
Ofloxacin, 70
Oncogenes, tyrosine kinase activity, 6
Opportunistic infections, AIDS, 85-95
Orciprenaline, obstructive airway diseases, 20
Osteoarthropathy, hypertrophic pulmonary (HPOA), 128
Otitis media, 73
Oxitropium bromide, 24
Oxygen therapy
  administration methods, 50, 51-54
  carbon dioxide retention, 63
  COAD, 43
  continuous positive pressure ventilation (CPAP), 51, 52
  domiciliary, long-term, 51-52, 53
  fixed performance devices, 51
  hypoxaemia in pneumonia, 78
  low-flow, 63
  oxygen concentrator, 52
  portable, 53-54
  respiratory failure, 51-54
  secondary pulmonary hypertension, 138
  short burst, 54
  transtracheal (TTO), 52-53
  variable performance devices, 51
Oxytetracycline, 70

# P

PAF antagonists, 46
Pain control, lung cancer, 126, 128-129
Palpitations, β-agonist-associated, 21
Para-aminosalicylic acid (PAS)
  adverse reactions, 105
  dosages, 98, 104
  in tuberculosis, 104-105
Paraneoplastic syndromes, lung

cancer, 127-128
Parenchymal pulmonary disease,
    drug-induced, 163-165
Parenteral therapy, 11
PCP see Pneumocystis carinii
    pneumonia (PCP)
PEEP, in ARDS, 145-146
Pellagra, isoniazid-related, 102
Penicillamine, SLE induction,
    lung effects, 164
Penicillin, V, 68
   pharyngitis, 73
Penicillin G, 68
Penicillins , 68-69
Pentamidine
   adverse reactions, 90
   nebulised
      cough/bronchospasm
        induction, 163
      in PCP, 91
        PCP prophylaxis, 94
   parenteral therapy, in PCP, 90
   versus co-trimoxazole, in PCP, 90
Pentoxifylline, 150
Pericardial effusions, tuberculous, 112
Pericarditis, traetment,
    in lung cancer, 129
Pharmacodynamics, 3-8
Pharmacokinetics, 1-3
Pharyngitis, 73
   diphtherial, 73
Phlebotomy, obstructive
    sleep apnoea, 64
Pholcodeine, 157-158
Phosphodiesterase (PDE) inhibition
   selective, 45-46
   theophylline, 26
Phosphoinostide (4, 5) biphosphate,
    hydrolysis, $CA^{2+}$ release, 6
Phospholipase $A_2$, inhibitions, 31, 46
Physiotherapy, in pneumonia, 78, 80
Pink puffers, 160
Piperacillin, 68
Pleural effusions, tuberculous, 112
Pneumocystis carinii pneumonia
    (PCP), AIDS, 85, 86, 89-93
   clinical features, 86-87
   deterioration, causes, 92
   prophylaxis, 94
Pneumonia, 73-81
   antibiotics, choice, 77-78, 79-81
   aspiration, 74, 75
      specific antibiotic therapy, 80-81
   bacterial
      in AIDS, 92-93
      causes, 74
      prevention, in AIDS, 94-95
   clinical approach, 74-76
   community-acquired, 74-75
      specific antibiotic therapy, 80

general investigation, 77
hospital-acquired, 74-75
   specific antibiotic therapy, 80
and host abnormalities, 78
in immunocompromised, 74, 75-76
   specific antibiotic therapy, 81
intensive care indications, 77
laboratory diagnosis, 76-77
specific antibiotic therapy, 79-81
supportive measures, 78, 80
therapeutic approach, 77-81
therapeutic response, 78
see also Pneumocystis carinii
    pneumonia (PCP)
Pneumonitis, gold-induced, 164
Potassium channel activators, 45
Potentiation, drugs, 8
Prednisolone, 30
   oral, absorption, 32-33
   plasma half-life, 33
Pregnancy, and antituberculosis
    drugs, 110-111
Procainamide, 165
Progestational hormones,
    respiratory stimulation, 56
Progesterone, premenstrual
    asthma, 42
Promethazine, 160
Propafenone, 44
Prostacyclin, in primary pulmonary
    hypertension, 136
Prostaglandin inhibition,
    theophylline, 27
Prostaglandins, in ARDS, 150
Prothionamide, in tuberculosis, 105
Protriptylline, 56
Protryptiline, sleep apnoea, 64
Pseudomembranous colitis,
    clindamycine-related, 71
Psittacosis, 74
Pulmonary artery occlusion pressure
    (PAOP), 132
Pulmonary disease, drug-related,
    160-165
Pulmonary embolus, 139, 141-145
   acute massive, 142, 143, 144-145
   acute minor, 142, 144
   chronic thromboembolic disease,
      142, 145
   surgery, 143-144
   therapy, 142-145
Pulmonary fibrosis, haemorrhagic, 119
Pulmonary vascular resistance
    (PVR), 131-132
Pyrazinamide
   adverse reactions, 103-104
   dosages, 98, 99, 103
   in tuberculosis, 103-104
Pyridoxine, in isoniazid peripheral
    neuropathy, 102

Q

Q fever, 74
Quinolones, 70-71

R

Radiation pneumonitis, and
    cyclophosphamide, 119
Radioligand binding, drug/
    receptor interaction, 4
Radiotherapy
   inoperable patients, 126
   non-small cell lung cancer (NSCLC),
      125-127, 129, 130
   palliative, 126-127
   postoperative, 125-126
   preoperative, 125
Rathadine, 105
Receptors
   drug interactions, 3-4
   fast, 6, 7
   slow, 6, 7
   types, 5
Red man syndrome, rifampicin
    overdosage, 100
Renal impairment, and
    antituberculosis drugs, 110
Respiratory diseases, causes, in
    immunocompromised, 76
Respiratory distress syndrome, adult
    see Adult respiratory distress
    syndrome (ARDS)
Respiratory failure
   classification, 49
   clinical patterns, 50
   diuretics, 57
   hypoxaemic, 62
   mucolytic agents, 54-55
   non-invasive mechanical
      ventilation, 57
   pathophysiology, therapy
      implications, 49-50
   pharmacotherapy, 50-58
   pure ventilatory, 62
   ventilatory/hypoxaemic, 62-63
      carbonic anhydrase
        inhibition, 56-57
   see also COPD; Cor pulmonale:
      Cor pulmonale
Respiratory infections see Infections,
    respiratory
Respiratory muscle fatigue, 57, 58-60
Respiratory stimulants, 63-64
   classification, 55
   COPD, 55-56
Retrobulbar neuritis, ethambutol-
    related, 102
Rhinitis, 72
Rifabutin, 105

Rifampicin
  adverse reactions, 100-101
  cutaneous reactions, 100
  dosages, 98, 99
  drug metabolic interactions, 101
  gastrointestinal reactions, 100
  and hepatic enzyme levels, 100, 101
  overdosage, red man syndrome, 100
  pharmacodynamics, 99
  pharmacokinetics, 99-100
  thrombocytopenic purpura, 100
  in tuberculosis, 98-101
Rifapentine, 105

## S

Salbutamol, 17, 63
SCLC *see* Small cell lung cancer (SCLC)
Second messengers, 4-7
Sedatives, contraindication in asthma, 44
Sepsis syndrome, inflammatory
        mediators, 148, 149
Sickle cell disease, 78
Sinusitis, 72
Sleep apnoea, 60-62
  body weight control, 61
  clinical presentation/diagnosis, 60-61
  nasal CPAP, 61-62, 64
  obstructive, 64
  pharmacotherapy, 61
  $SaO_2$ measurement, 61
  tracheostomy, 62
  types, 60
  upper airway obstruction, 61, 64
Small cell lung cancer (SCLC)
  chemotherapy, 121-124
    combination regimens, 122
    duration, 123-124
    efficacy studies, 123-124
    maintenance, 123, 124
    and quality of life, 123-124
    response/survival rates, 122
  growth rate, 117
  long-term survival parameters, 124
Sodium aurothiomalate, pulmonary
        fibrosis induction, 164
Sodium cromoglycate (SCG), 36-37
  administration, 36
  clinical use, 36-37
  mode of action, 36
  *pKa*, 2
  side-effects, 36
Spacer chambers, inhaled drugs, 10
Spironolactone, in cor pulmonale, 57
Steroid receptors, 31
Steroids
  in ARDS, 148-149
  *see also* Corticosteroids;
  Glucocorticoid receptors *and* therapy
Strammonium, 23
*Streptococcus pneumoniae*, COAD, 43

Streptokinase, in pulmonary
        embolus, 143
Streptomycin
  adverse reactions, 103
  8th cranial nerve damage, 103
  dosages, 98, 99, 103
  in tuberculosis, 102-103
Sulphamethoxazole-trimethoprim *see*
        Co-trimoxazole
Surfactant, in ARDS, 151
Sympathomimetic amines, respiratory
        muscle fatigue, 58-59
Synergism, drugs, 8

## T

Tachycardia, β-agonist-associated, 21
Tachyphylaxis, 8
Taste, ipratropium bromide effects on, 25
Terbutaline, 17
  in respiratory muscle fatigue, 58-59
Tetracyclines, 70
Theophylline
  action, 27
  administration routes, 28-29
  chemistry, 26
  clearance, affecting factors, 28
  clinical use, 29-30
  in COAD, 43
  drug interactions, 2-3
  intravenous, 28
  mode of action, 26-27
  obstructive airway diseases, 25-30
  oral, 28-29
  pharmacokinetics, 27-28
  in respiratory muscle fatigue, 58
  respiratory stimulation, 55-56
  side-effects, 29
  Vd, 2
Thiacetazone
  adverse reactions, 104
  dosages, 99, 104
  in tuberculosis, 104
Thrombocytopenic purpura,
        rifampicin-related, 100
Thromboembolic disease
  chronic, 142, 145
  definition, 139
  epidemiology, 139-140
Thrombolysis
  in deep venous thrombosis, 141
  in pulmonary embolus, 143
Thromboxane antagonists, 46
Ticarcillin, 68
Tobramycin, 69
Tocainide, 165
Tolerance, drugs, 8
Tracheostomy
  sleep apnoea, 62
  *see also* Minitracheostomy
Transbronchial biopsy, PCP

diagnosis, 87-88
Transtracheal oxygen
        (TTO) therapy, 52-53
  complications, 53
Triamcinolone
  acetonide, structure, 30
  steroid-resistant asthma, 42
Tricyclic antidepressants, respiratory
        stimulation, 56
Trimethoprim-sulphamethoxazole
        *see* Co-trimoxazole
Trimetrexate, in PCP, 91
Tuberculosis
  chemoprophylaxis, 113-114
  drug therapy
    aims, 107
    daily dosages, 98
    failure, 109-110, 113
    intermittent dosages, 99
    regimen choice, 108-110
    *see also* Antituberculosis drugs
  drugs list, 98
  epidemiology, 97-98
  extrapulmonary, chemotherapy,
        111-112
  in immunosuppressed, 111
  newly diagnosed patients,
        drug regimens, 108
  notifications increase, 97
  prevention, in AIDS, 94
Tyrosine kinase, 6

## U

Upper airway obstruction,
        sleep apnoea, 61, 64
Upper respiratory tract infections,
        71-73
  bacterial pathogens, 72
Urokinase, in pulmonary embolus, 143
Uvulopalatopharyngoplasty
        (UVPPP), 64

## V

Vancomycin, 71
Vascular disease, pulmonary, 131
Vasodilators, 138
  adverse effects, 136, 138
  primary pulmonary
        hypertension, 135-137
  secondary pulmonary
        hypertension, 138
Vena caval filter
  in deep venous thrombosis, 141
  in pulmonary embolus, 144
Ventilation, new modes, in
        ARDS, 146-147

Ventilatory support, new
   approaches, 145-146
Ventimask, oxygen therapy, 51
Vinblastine, 120
Vinca alkaloids, in lung cancer, 120
Vincristine, 120
Vindesine, 120

**W**

Warfarin, in deep venous
   thrombosis, 141
Wegener's granulomatosis, 116

**Z**

Zidovudine (AZT), 86, 87
   adverse reactions, 88
   anti-retroviral treatment, in HIV
      infection, 87-88
Zinc fingers, 6